SuperSlaw

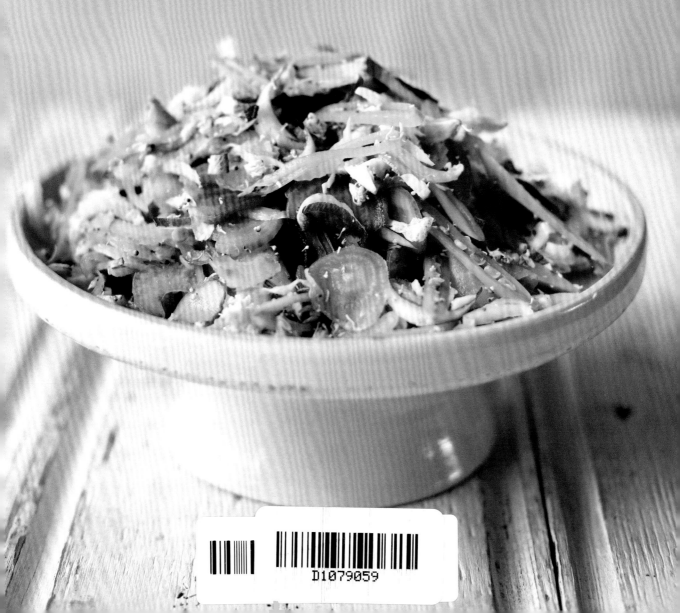

10 9 8 7 6 5 4 3 2 1

Ebury Press, an imprint of Ebury Publishing,
20 Vauxhall Bridge Road,
London, SW1V 2SA

Ebury Press is part of the Penguin Random House group of companies whose addresses can be found at
global.penguinrandomhouse.com

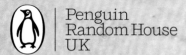

Penguin
Random House
UK

First published by Ebury Press in 2017

www.penguin.co.uk

A CIP catalogue record for this book is available from the British Library

Design: Barbara Zúñiga
Photography: Lara Messer
Food and Prop Styling: Frankie Unsworth
Copy-edit: Kay Halsey
Nutritional read: Kerry Torrens
Index: Vanessa Bird
Production: Helen Everson

ISBN: 978-1-785-03554-8

Printed and bound in China by C&C Offset Co Ltd

The nutrition and health claims made in this book have all been checked by a registered food nutritionist.

Penguin Random House is committed to a sustainable future for our business, our readers and our planet.
This book is made from Forest Stewardship Council® certified paper.

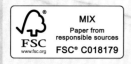

SuperSlaw

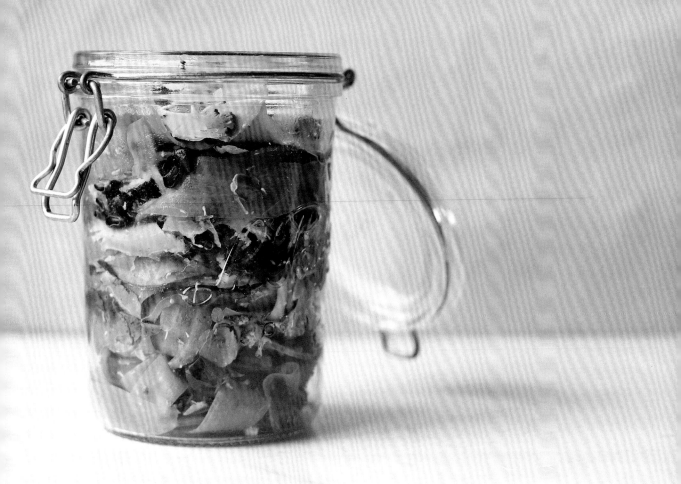

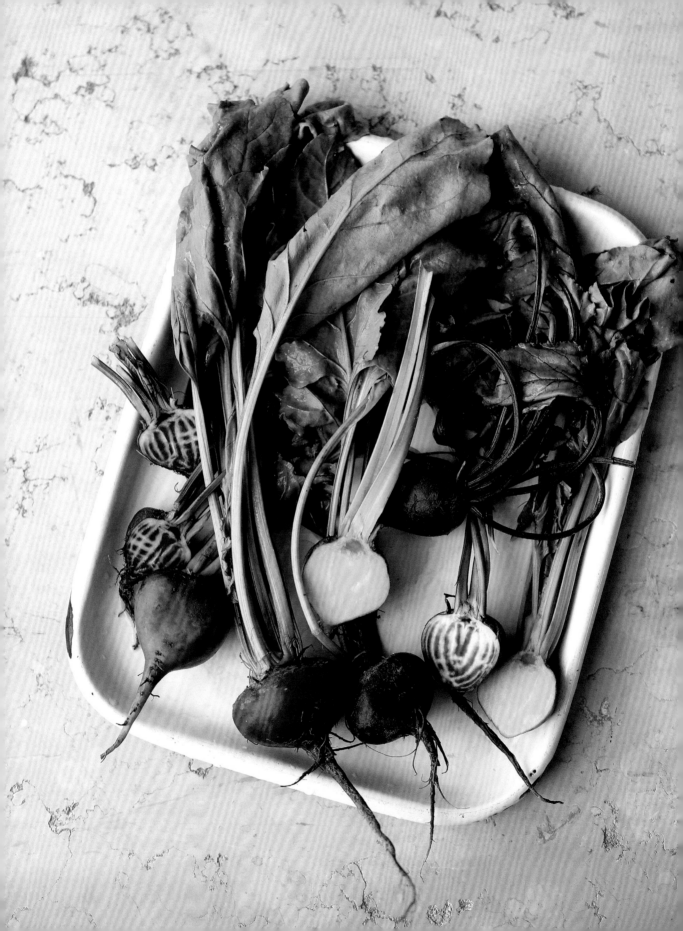

Contents

Creation of #SuperSlaw 6

What is SuperSlaw 10

SuperSlaw Essentials 14

Hydrolyze 22

Immunity 42

Energy Booster 66

Revitalize 88

Recovery 112

Thermic + Spicy 132

Additional Recommendations for Macronutrients 156

Index 158

Acknowledgements 160

The creation of #SuperSlaw

Opening a near empty fridge after work one night I noticed a common theme had emerged.

Firstly, I had returned home after a long day at work, feeling like a women possessed, with food rage. Food rage is an acute condition, leading to anyone or anything standing in the way of the fridge being at risk of possible severe harm. Sensible and

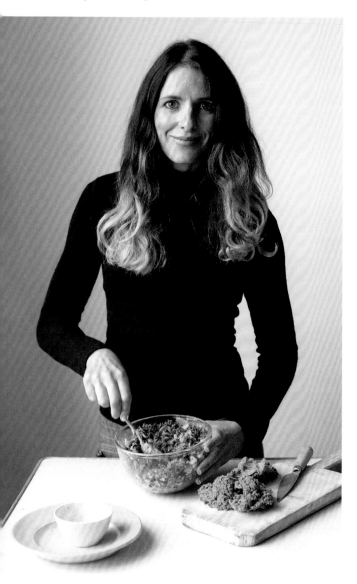

balanced food choices at a time of 'H-anger' are a challenge. Fellow sufferers may empathise when I say that in moments of food rage the family pet sometimes starts to look appealing as a side order — with extra fries. At times of such uncertainty in our blood sugars, our mind tends not to be our own, and the rational decision to take time out and prepare some healthy vegetables to meet our clean living, five-a-day targets is unlikely to happen thanks to the symptoms of irritability, mood swings and total irrationality that have taken us over. This is never a great time to nip to the local shops. You will return with most of the supermarket, but probably nothing that actually constitutes a full and balanced meal.

Secondly, I found myself bored by the requirement to prepare a meal so it covered the full range of nutrients that my body needed. I had reached crisis point. I had become stuck in a veggie rut, using the same monotonous vegetables and salads each night, through pure habit and a lack of imagination. I was bored by five-a-day. I wanted something new. Steamed kale and broccoli no longer hit the spot for vegetable excitement. I needed to act.

As a personal trainer I advise my clients to try and prepare their meals in advance, but as I also have a second job that involves work in front of a computer for very long hours, I know what it's like to struggle to find healthy choices whilst stuck in an office. To make it even harder, prepping veggies and salads seemed to be a dull and laborious task. I noticed my fitness clients often ended up filling lunch boxes with expensive green powders, bored with the peeling and chopping of mundane salads or carrot batons. What we all lacked was time and inspiration.

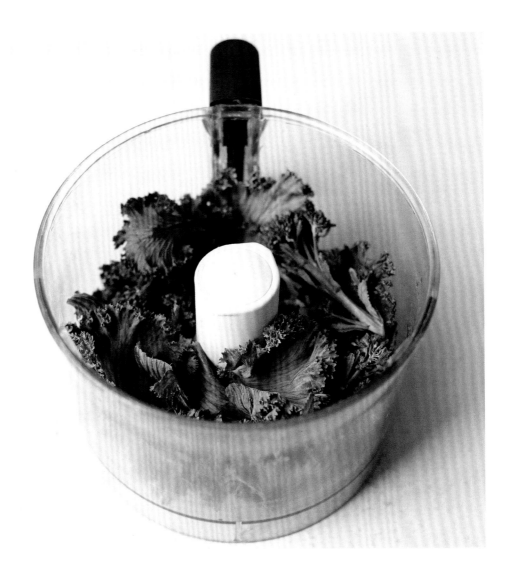

How else could we plan and prepare interesting vegetables ahead of time without it being laborious?

So, returning to my food rage moment, with a need for extra nutrition, a few green veggies sitting alone in my fridge and a lack of time and patience to prepare, a light bulb moment struck. Noticing my food processor gathering dust in my kitchen cupboard, I thought how could I create an easier method of mixing my greens into a healthful meal? I began experimenting by chopping away with haste. I soon found myself using condiments, herbs and spices that would otherwise have remained untouched in my kitchen. Supermarket shopping became more vegetable focused and recipe requests soon started flowing.

Introducing the concept of SuperSlaw to clients and fellow coaches scored an overwhelming victory for those who needed extra vitamins from the stress placed on their bodies following endurance-based or extreme training schedules. Those who were looking for extra fibre or greens for a fat-loss plan were also excited by the ease at which SuperSlaw could be added into everyday meals.

This was the moment SuperSlaw was born. It was a solution to my troubles. I hope it will now be a solution for you too.

How SuperSlaw will make you healthy and happy

Health is often defined as the absence of disease. One of the biggest problems with health is that we overlook it, taking it for granted until one day it starts to fail. Signs and symptoms of disease begin to show. Usually at this point we lean on the medical profession for drugs and quick-fix solutions so that we can get back to our superfast life with the same ferocity. Others may send themselves off to the latest detox camp for a week of self loathing, living off a bowl of cabbage, committed to a life of repentance – until the next social event calls and they are back to square one! Tiredness is seen as normality. Energy is seen as something that happens in a gym or following a caffeinated drink.

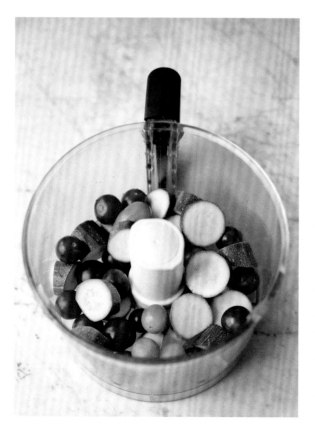

A key point about good health is the relationship this area has with happiness and contentment. You'd be hard pushed to find someone who is suffering with stress, anxiety and depression, but who also appears full of vitality and looks a picture of glowing health. Health and happiness are interconnected. This is why when our diet is unhealthy, void of proper nutrition, or loaded with chemicals, we get mood fluctuations.

Have you ever fed a child a giant bag of multicoloured sweets? I am willing to bet you will see a change in their mood that is not usually restaurant-friendly. Have you ever grabbed a quick pick-me-up (in the form of the same bag of sweets)? What did you notice about your energy in the aftermath? My guess is a stimulated synthetic fix, followed by a low-level mood slump. Am I close?

Conversely, when our diet is rich in vitamins and minerals, research suggests there can be a positive mood change and a stable supply of energy. Our skin, hair, nails and personalities begin to glow. Medical treatments now increasingly look to diet as an essential aspect of treating severe health-related conditions. Ask anyone who has ever suffered with high blood pressure or a gout attack what the first thing their GP asked them about and diet will be top of the list.

Hormones are pivotal in driving our mood and food plays a key role in driving our hormones. It's all a cycle of chemical reaction, that's just how the body works. What we eat influences our mood and thereby influences our overall happiness. It is increasingly up to us to manage our own health through good nutrition. So, as busy as we are, we need to handle it.

The best nutrition plan for health and happiness?

If I had the answer to this question I would be up for a Nobel nutrition peace prize. There are infinite responses, theories and diet books that profess their nutritional approach is the best way to slim down or gain energy or become a brighter, tighter human being.

The 'low-carb, paleo, raw, clean eating, low-fat, SIRT, high-carb' diet guides (to name just a few) all provide in part legitimate and sustainable eating plans and pointers for most people. Those who follow their approaches often find hard-and-fast results for a diverse range of health goals, and this is despite the seeming contradictions and disagreements amongst the macronutrient principles and content. Some argue fat is bad, others argue eat more fat. Whilst carbs have been given a bad reputation over the last few years (see paleo), others argue that carbs should fill most of our plates! Some say starch is in. For others starch is out. Even government guidance is contradictory, dependant upon what country you live in! It's no wonder we get confused.

I'm a believer in personal experimentation. Having worked with this philosophy, however,

I have also found there is no one size fits all approach, nothing that works for every person. What works well for someone with a high carbohydrate tolerance who is very active, will not necessarily work the same for the person who is sedentary and overweight. Female hormones can alter how they use fuel. At different times of the menstrual cycle even the body may respond better to fats than carbohydrates, and vice versa at other times of the month (sorry chaps), when carbohydrates seem to come out on top. Stress changes hormones and again can influence how the body uses (or fails to use in certain cases) different sources of fuel. This is why two people following exactly the same diet or exercise plan can often achieve very different results. People have different goals, bodies and physiologies. They also have different hormones depending on their lifestyles. We are all unique. However, what I have begun to find most interesting in all of the existing nutritional plans is not what is different about each nutritional recommendation, but what is the same.

What do almost all diet or nutritional plans have in common?

Regardless of the craziness of some of the health plans I have seen, having researched this issue for numerous years, vegetables seem to come out on top as being the most consistent feature of any nutritional health-related programme. Even in the strictest of plans that ban fruit, vegetables will feature in some form or another.

In terms of importance in almost every health buff's tool kit, vegetables will come out on top. This is not to say that I am encouraging a solely vegetarian diet. Regardless of whether the veggies are paired with meat, fish or tofu, they are consistently flagged as the golden key to health, regardless of your goal.

What is SuperSlaw?

SuperSlaw recipes are all founded on a nutritiously dense base of micro-chopped vegetables. I devised the concept of SuperSlaw as a way to quickly prepare hot and cold nutritionally balanced meals that put the vegetables first, and also didn't require me to invest extra time and effort in the kitchen.

Whatever the latest eating craze, experts agree that by increasing the quota of vegetables in your diet you will increase your strength, health and happiness. There will always be a new approach to eating. These usually begin in January with a sense of self-gratification and a bit of a buzz over the exciting start of a new journey, with mental images of a trim body cleansed from the inside out. Then by the end in March, when the regime becomes tiresome and perhaps too expensive and time consuming, the cold, hard truth and less glamorous reality hits home: extreme quick-fix solutions to health rarely lead to long-term change, and old habits tend to stubbornly creep back in.

Working as a personal trainer and nutrition advisor for many years, trying multiple diets and eating plans, I have come to realize the way to change our eating habits is to focus not on restricting foods, but on including foods, and not on radical, intensive change, but on habit change — gradually sneaking highly nutritious foods into our daily routine, leaving less room (and ultimately less desire) for foods with low nutritional value. SuperSlaw enables this more sustainable approach, and into the bargain it also saves you money, effort and time — more time to gloat over the multiple health benefits of the new health kick you are about to introduce.

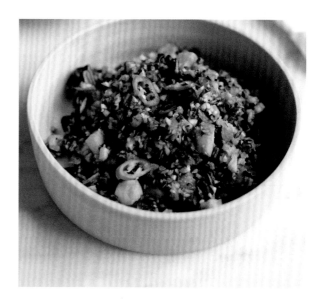

Whether cooking for one or for a family, SuperSlaw will help you make simple, long-term healthful changes to your diet by adding in an increased portion of vegetables each day in a new, exciting way. What's more, each recipe comes with ideas on how to MORPH your highly nutritious SuperSlaw base into a hot meal and how to add TOPPERS to your SuperSlaw, including adding macronutrients, powering up its taste and nutritional value.

Life seems to get faster and busier, creating an ever increasing need for convenience. As Leonardo Da Vinci once said, 'Simplicity is the ultimate sophistication,' and I am about to share with you how to turn what some may consider mundane, everyday veggies into delicious, nutritious rainbow food. Life is demanding and although I think we sometimes like it that way, the unwanted consequence of busyness is the impact on our health. SuperSlaw fits easily into the busiest of routines to change how you live, look and feel.

SuperFast

Most SuperSlaws take a few minutes to prepare using a food processor, but are still quick if you prefer to prepare by hand with a knife, chopping board, spiralizer or mandolin. They involve hardly any weighing, measuring or calculating.

SuperVersatile

SuperSlaws can be served as a snack, a dessert, a side portion, a packed lunch, morphed into another meal, topped with macronutrients, added to other dishes, eaten raw or cooked.

SuperConvenient

No need to hunt for unusual ingredients in specialist shops. The recipes of SuperSlaw involve easily sourced vegetables and readily available cupboard ingredients. They can be prepared last minute or ahead of time for meals based around a full, healthy plate of macronutrients. If prepared ahead, they also serve as a healthy option on standby in case of a snack attack.

SuperResourceful

SuperSlaws avoid waste by experimenting, adding from your existing food stock or leftovers, as mixers, TOPPERS or MORPHS, or add some of your SuperSlaw mix to other meals for additional nutrients and fibre.

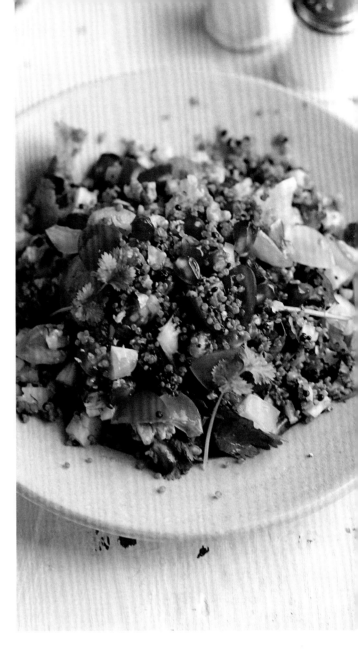

SuperTasty

SuperSlaws make vegetables fun, more tasty and endlessly varied – a great way to introduce more vegetables to the diets of veggie-phobics and fussy eaters. They don't involve complex preparation or obscure ingredients and will help you think outside the box about how you combine nutritionally dense foods for convenience and new tastes. These recipes are all made with fresh vegetables, herbs and spices or widely available cupboard ingredients.

SuperHealthy

SuperSlaws are a mass of vitamins and minerals, helping you meet fibre and micronutrient targets with ease. Each SuperSlaw has been developed with individual health benefits in mind, allowing you to pick and choose according to energy requirements and the busyness of your lifestyle. The bulk of any SuperSlaw is made predominantly from vegetables, and they encourage the use of natural ingredients wherever possible.

The case for chewing rather than drinking your fruit and veg

Juices and smoothies are a fantastic way of introducing a quick nutritional blast for most health-conscious people. However, there is some often overlooked food for thought in the world of juices.

Firstly, juicing fruit and vegetables basically means you don't have to chew. From an evolutionary standpoint, most researchers agree that teeth allowed humans (or cave men) to tear and break down tough food in the mouth. Dental experts advocate chewing as a way of maintaining good dental health, as the movement itself encourages strong jaw development. Saliva created by chewing also helps remineralise the teeth and acid balance in the mouth, whilst its digestive enzymes help to break down some of the carbohydrates and fats found in food even before they leave the mouth. Chewing therefore aids digestion and starts this process in the mouth.

Secondly, juicing foods reduces fibre. For most healthy people, encouraging the body to process fibre in food is a pivotal part of what is considered to be a good digestive system flow. Foods with a lower fibre content can lead to us lacking in the wonderful feeling of fullness. This is why you can drink a juice in seconds and often still feel hungry as the straw hits the bottom of the glass! Fibre:

- Provides 'fuel' to support good bacteria growth.
- Helps control your blood sugar levels.
- Contributes to lowering cholesterol.
- Regulates the movement of food through the digestive tract. We need food to digest at the correct rate or it can seriously impact on our energy levels. This is 'sluggish digestion'.
- Helps maintain health of the digestive tract.

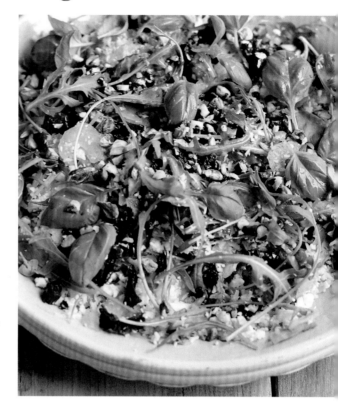

Good digestive health helps control when you feel full, and when you feel hungry. This plays a huge role in how well we manage our overall diet and if, and how, we get lean and feel satiated. Good digestive health also needs to take place at the correct rate to allow nutrients and minerals time to be absorbed.

A sluggish digestive system can lead to weight gain and many other much more serious health-related problems. You may not be getting what you pay for on a diet that focuses for nutrition purposes entirely on juicing. Juices taste great. My advice is drink them as you wish, but try and include them in your diet as an addition to five-a-day targets and other real foods, not as your main source of nutrition.

The case for a veggie-based diet

- Vegetables are rich in fibre.
- Most vegetables, and especially green vegetables, help sustain healthy blood sugar levels, and healthy blood sugar levels mean stable mood and stable energy levels.
- Vegetables are low in calories. It is very hard to overeat on most vegetables, so the good news is you can stock up without having to worry about calorie counting or weight gain.
- Vegetables provide an endless supply of vitamins and minerals. Vitamins and minerals are needed by the body to stay strong and healthy. When the body lacks the vitamins and minerals it needs, it will not function in the way it is supposed to, creating an environment primed for ill-health and fatigue.
- Vegetables hold an abundance of phytonutrients. Phytonutrients are the superpower chemicals found in plants linked to the prevention of many diseases.
- Due to the extensive range of vitamins and minerals found in vegetables, they contribute to slowing down the ageing process. As we know, healthy eating is more often than not evidenced through our skin.
- Vegetables are important for the promotion of good gut health. Many recent studies have identified the importance of certain raw vegetables serving as pre-biotics in the gut. While probiotics introduce good bacteria, pre-biotics encourage the expansion of the much needed good-bad bacteria ratio. Good gut health is known to relate to superior health.

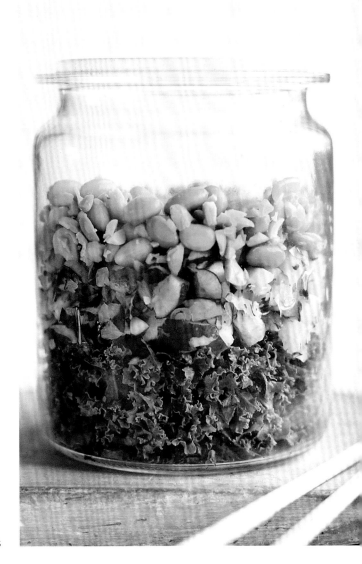

- Vegetables are easy to buy or grow. From a box or patch in your own back garden to superstores, farm shops, markets or greengrocers.
- Vegetables are natural.

SuperSlaw Essentials

What ingredients do I need to make a SuperSlaw?

Fruits /Vegetables/Fresh herbs This is the 'bulk of the slaw'. I recommend organic wherever possible, however, the target with a SuperSlaw is to add as much of your five-a-day into your diet as you can. So if you need to use peas from the freezer or vegetables in a packet from your local supermarket to make life easier, then work with what you have and what you can afford (for non-organic produce just ensure you wash any ingredients thoroughly before use). SuperSlaw is all about convenience.

Olive oil Always buy extra virgin and the best quality oil you can afford.

Vinegar Red, white, balsamic and cider. Again, go for the best quality of vinegar that you can afford.

Condiments Many of our dressings will include an added spice or flavour from a range of sauces or condiments, most of which you probably already stock in your family kitchen. Examples are horseradish, mustard (Dijon, wholegrain, French), mint, tahini, apple, relishes, pickles, cranberry and chilli. Depending on the quality and brand of the product you use, this may increase the sugar content of the slaw. However, the amounts recommended within the recipe will make this marginal.

Sea salt Unrefined salt contains many helpful minerals that the body can use to promote good health, whilst refined table salt is heavily processed and the processing limits any benefits for the body. Sea salt and rock salt are great examples of minimally processed salts, which make a super addition to any slaw. Buy the best you can afford, and experiment with the different varieties on offer.

Spices Some recipes will contain spices that you may or may not have in your cupboard. A good spice rack is a welcome addition to give any slaw an extra kick.

Nuts/Seeds For those who tolerate nuts and seeds well, the added benefit of extra good fats and a bit of crunch is a SuperSlaw bonus. Nuts and seeds are known to go 'rancid' (off) quickly, so keep your nuts tip-top by storing in a sealed airtight container. One of my personal favourite places to store nuts is the freezer, which keeps them extra crunchy and extra fresh.

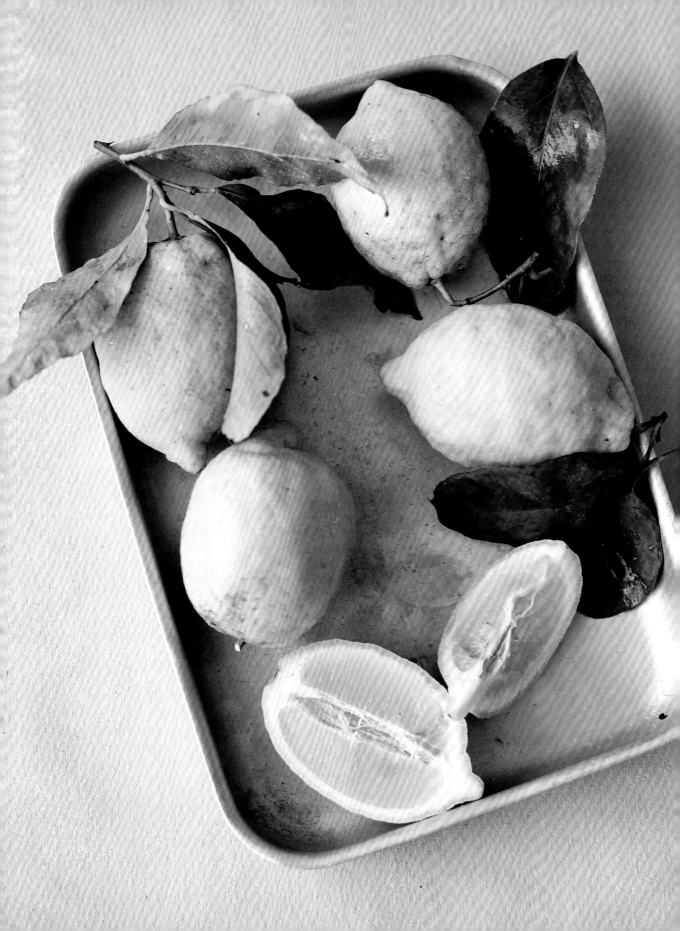

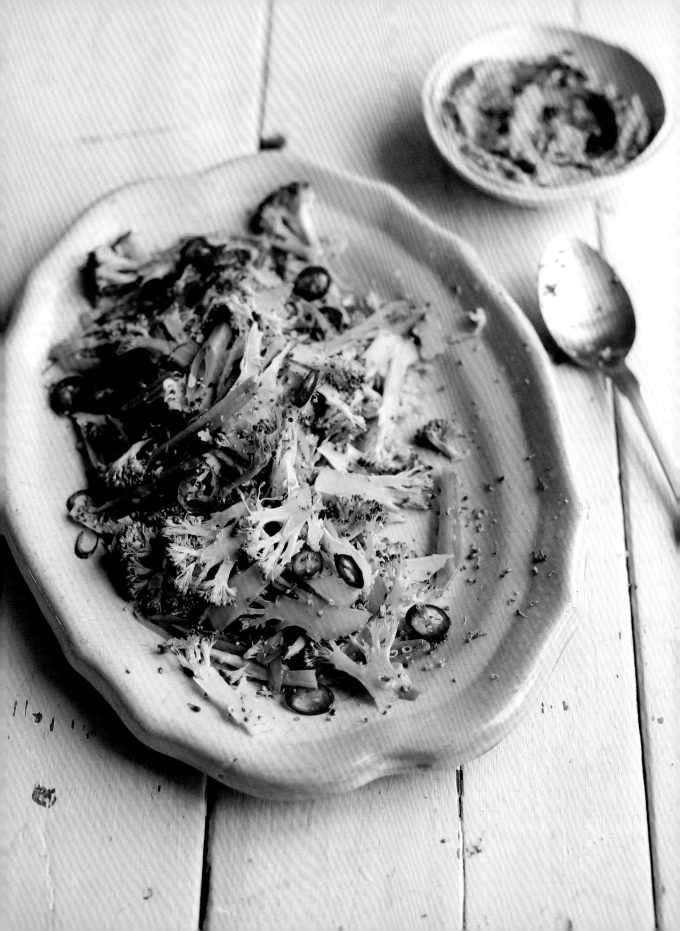

What equipment do I need to make a SuperSlaw?

Sharp knife A sharp knife is helpful for any topping and tailing and the removal of the core. If you don't own a food processor then the complete slaw can also be chopped by hand. You can experiment with the coarseness and thickness of the vegetables if you have a good knife selection but, if you don't, a good chef's knife (generally 20 cm) is a must-have for efficient chopping.

Peeler A good-quality peeler can be used to peel the skin from vegetables, although you may prefer to scrub the veg. Wider peelers can be used to create a ribbon effect if you want a more decorative SuperSlaw. The secret to a good peeler not only lies in the sharpness of the blade, but also the comfort and grip of the handle, so look out for this as well.

Spiralizer Spiralizers add a beautifully decorative addition to any SuperSlaw, and there are heaps of options on the market these days with a range of tool adaptations. Spiralizers create a curly ribbon effect, best used on dense or harder veggies. If you are super keen on the spiralizer effect, then my advice is to look at investing in a larger 'stand-alone' tool, as they seem to be more efficient and less time consuming if you wish to prepare a slaw in bulk.

Grater A grater is helpful for creating a fine zest from any citrus fruit or an easy addition of garlic or ginger, which are often a little fiddly to chop.

Mandolin Fabulous for helping achieve a decorative 'julienne' (long strip) or more uniform slice by hand.

Food processor If you have never experienced a food processor before, you have nothing to fear as long as you learn how to put the lid on correctly! I use a food processor for ease and convenience. It saves heaps of time and enables you to make SuperSlaw in bulk.

If you own a food processor and use it infrequently, now is the time to take it out of the cupboard and start to store it as a functional piece of visual kitchen equipment on your worktop. This will encourage you to use it more regularly.

I use a food processor for most of my recipes for speed. Because I prepare almost all of my slaws in bulk, I make large amounts and store them in the fridge ready to throw into meals or serve as a side.

If you don't have a food mixer or prefer to use a knife, spiralizer, grater or mandolin, you can. It will take a little longer, but taste just as good. Dependent upon the method used, the appearance of the slaw may differ. In this book we have used a variety of chopping methods to show you the variations that are possible.

Large storage container And/or lots of smaller containers are useful to aid meal preparation throughout the week.

Jam jar with a lid Used for mixing dressings.

Large mixing or salad bowl

Large mixing spoon

Chopping board

Preparation tips for making a SuperSlaw

Veggie chopping

The chopping blades on a food processor are changeable and I vary the blades I use to give different textures to my slaw. For a smaller, chunkier cut, the central blade that inserts into the bottom of the main bowl is usually the best chopper and the one I use most often. Be prepared if you have a 'superfast' food processor as this can often lead to a very fine consistency, so test this out. Dependant on the model of your food processor, the settings may or may not include multiple speed settings.

Favour a light, brief pulsing or clicking action on the button (on and off very quickly), as opposed to holding your finger down; get to know your machine.

Alternatively, for a more traditional style of slaw, the flat chopper blade that fits closer to the lid (with the ingredients fed through the hole at the top) will give a flatter cut to your slaw. The blades will often have written instructions inscribed on each side, so have a look to check any guidance given. If a blade is reversible, it may give an indication of the coarseness of the chop it will provide.

Finally, avoid 'mushing' the vegetables together (unless the recipe says otherwise). Blend the slaw until the ingredients are finely chopped, but not so they are mushy. You want crunch from your slaw. Be aware that some veg, generally the harder veg, will take longer to chop than others. However, this still take seconds to do. Just press or pulse the processor button until you have 'chopped' and not 'mushed' your vegetables. If you find large chunks, this may be a sign you are overfilling the food processor. Simply pick out the larger pieces and throw back in to re-chop and, in future, add in batches.

Raw or cooked?

Most of the vegetables and herbs are placed in the food processor raw. However, on occasion a recipe may instruct you to place the ingredients into boiling or cold water to blanch for seconds first. This is the only 'cooking' that you will do. However, all slaws can be eaten hot or cold after preparation.

Dressings

After the chopping has taken place, mix your dressing vigorously in an empty jam jar. This enables the oil, vinegar and condiment to combine evenly and avoids separation. Pour the dressing over your slaw and check to see if the slaw is fully coated. This allows the slaw to keep in the fridge well. Any leftover dressing can be stored in the fridge ready for your next slaw creation. I love generous amounts of olive oil and vinegar in my slaws. Olive oil and good-quality vinegars have heaps of health benefits and also help preserve for longer. This is the same for any addition of lemon, lime or sea salt.

In this book

The recipe instructions all include the very simplest method of preparing your SuperSlaw and the most convenient way to create them using a food processor. However, they can all be completely or partially hand chopped using a knife, mandolin or spiraliser. We have pictured some of the various ways that you can hand chop to inspire you to try different methods, although all of the instructions will be on how to food process. There aren't strict methods, so feel free to chop and blitz as desired!

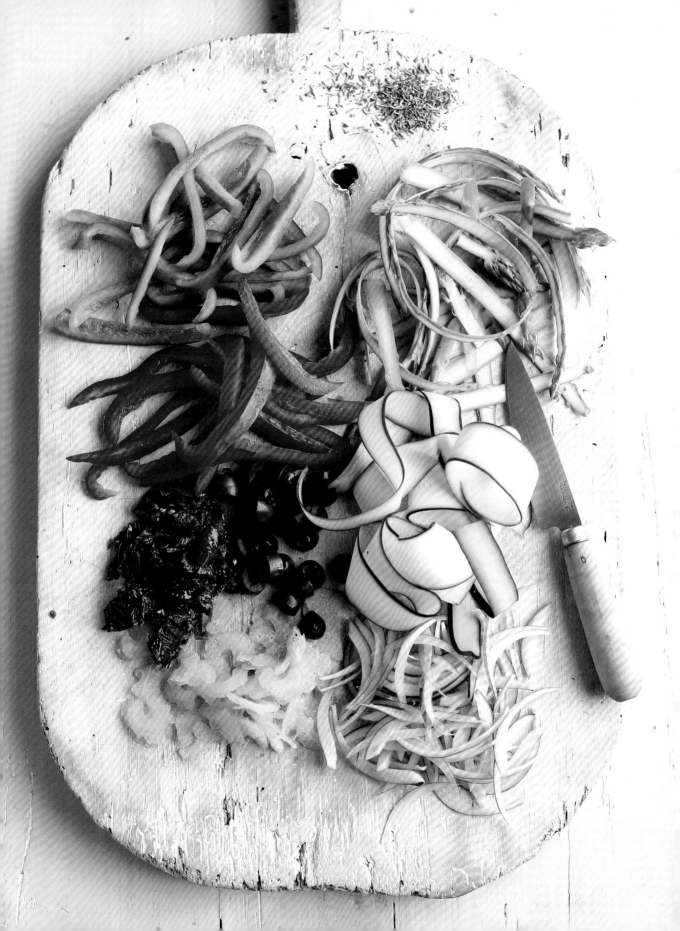

Serving your SuperSlaw

SuperSlaws are aimed to enrich daily diets with large portions of good vegetables and fruit. They can be served on their own as a snack or as a main meal.

SuperSlaws taste good any day, any time and no fixed rules apply to how and when you should eat them. I have, however, divided the recipes with some special SuperSlaw power labels according to their individual benefits, which should give you some guidance about serving suggestions in terms of your day-to-day individual needs.

In order to hit other macronutrient targets (fuels needed to promote energy, growth and repair), I have also given some recommendations of how to serve each slaw with a good-quality fat, protein and/ or starchy carbohydrate. This will help create a full and balanced meal.

Amounts of protein and carbohydrate recommendations will vary dependant on your individual goals. However, SuperSlaws are low in calories and as such you can generally eat as much of them as you wish regardless of your diet, nutrition or health plan.

TOPPERS

These are recommended to be used as a sprinkled topping at the end of preparation. Generally these are items that are best hand-chopped or kept whole.

MORPHS

Suggestions for MORPHS are included with each recipe and provide ideas of how you can easily use your slaw within other dishes. Eating a combination of raw and heated slaws is recommended for a greater diversity and maximum health benefits.

Most of our slaws, if dressed and stored well, will last for a few days at a time. I tend to make two very large SuperSlaws a week. Two large slaws will last two people to add to most meals for a seven-day period. Slaws can be eaten hot or cold and can MORPH into other recipes as an extra treat.

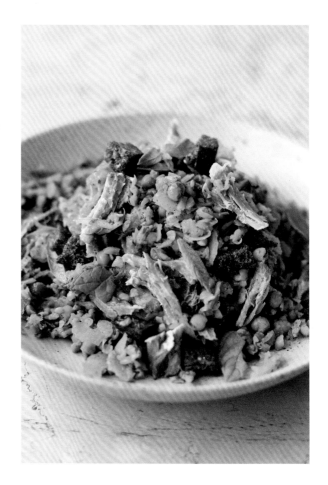

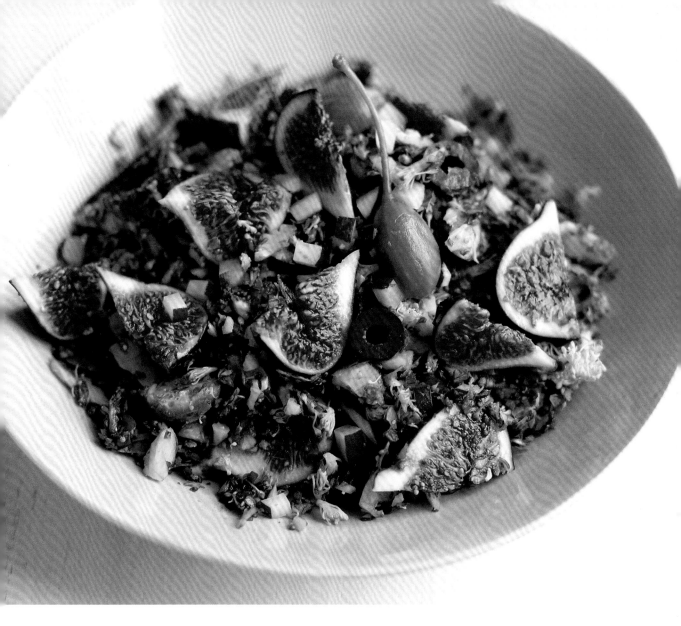

SuperSlaw: When does food become Super?

For me, keeping food simple, natural and nutrient dense wherever possible is the best philosophy and how I approach eating for health. SuperSlaw is based on this concept, ensuring you increase your five-a-day target with ease. With that in mind, however, it's well worth a mention that you will find all of the recipes hold multiple benefits. So whether you are a lover of superfoods, juicing, eating raw or following a vegetarian diet, you will find that SuperSlaws are a brilliant addition to your meal plans, as they will work perfectly amongst these disciplines.

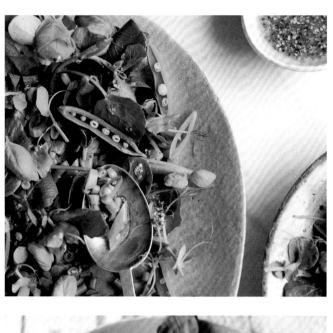

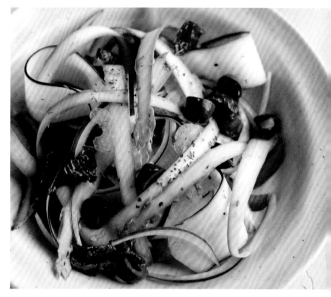

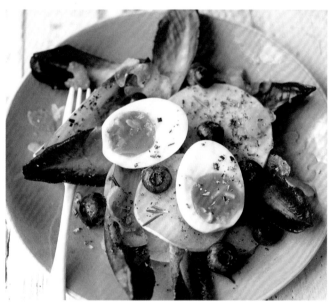

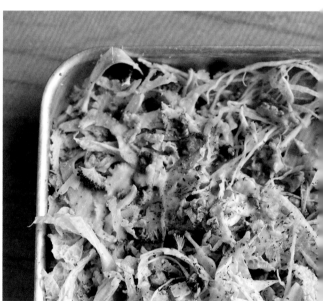

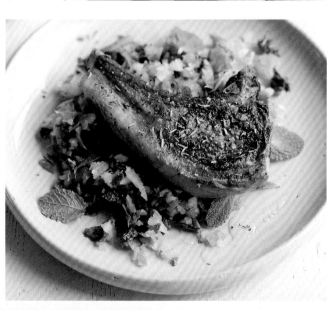

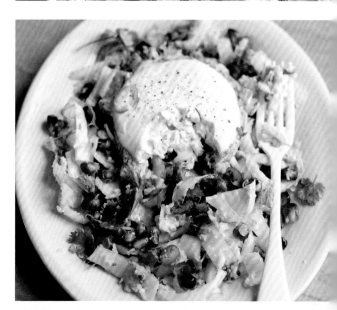

Hydrolyze

Maintaining a balance between the amounts of acid and alkaline foods you eat is a great guideline from a nutrition perspective. Some proponents say we should only eat alkaline foods, but this overlooks the nutritional benefits of some healthy food options, such as meat, grains or dairy, which are known to be acidic. More recent research regarding the alkaline-acid food debate indicates that both alkaline and acidic foods are beneficial for good health, and science is ongoing about the truth behind how foods that are said to be alkaline or acidic truly impact on PH levels within the body. The main conclusions seem to indicate that the inevitable increase in green vegetables that coincides with an alkaline diet (regardless of the truth behind the PH impact), from a health viewpoint will always be beneficial due to the increased density of nutrition. As always, 'balance' seems to be the key, so mixing in some meat or cheese with your veggies is a way to achieve this. Hydrolyze SuperSlaws work on the principle of balance, including high levels of green vegetables and TOPPERS or MORPHS, which include grains, protein and dairy.

A diet high in processed foods is not only said to be acidic, but can have a dehydrating effect on your body. The body is made up of roughly 60 per cent water and with a lack of regular rehydration, cells, organs and tissue can easily begin to decline in function. Water is lost through obvious processes, such as sweating or digestion. However, even breathing and ill health can lead to excess water being lost from the body. Luckily we can increase our water consumption by eating watery foods and Hydrolyze SuperSlaws were created using vegetables known for having a high water content. Great for anyone who forgets to drink enough or if you need a little extra hydration after a fun-filled weekend or workout.

Hydrolyze SuperSlaws also tend to be the slaw lowest in calories, so are great to pair with higher fat foods for those wanting to balance macronutrients. Alternatively, they work really well as a vitamin-rich, satiating but low-calorie snack.

Lively Lemon Slaw

I love lemons. When I was younger I went through a lemon stage, eating whole lemons whenever I could get my hands on them. Lemons are well reported to aid digestion, while also providing an alkalizing effect once inside the body. Often referred to as the Botox of the fruit bowl, lemons help prevent fruits or veggies turning brown, so your SuperSlaw will stay looking fresh. Perfect if you need to create a slaw for the following day.

1 head (400 g) of broccoli, cut into
   quarters
2 handfuls of flat-leaf parsley
2 handfuls of coriander
2 large spring onions (or 3 if they
   have small bulbs)
2 lemons, peeled and deseeded
1–2 tablespoons sumac
Sea salt
Drizzle of olive oil

Makes 4 large portions

TOPPER pictured

1 Place the central chopping attachment into the main bowl of the food processor.

2 Place the broccoli in the bowl and replace the lid.

3 Pulse it, in short bursts, into small, chunky pieces. Don't use the continuous pulse button or your mixture will be too fine.

4 Tip the broccoli into a waiting bowl.

5 Add the herbs, spring onions and fully peeled lemons to the food processor. Don't worry about mashing the lemons, they will mix into the slaw, creating a fantastically bold flavour. Pulse until chopped, then tip out over the chopped broccoli and stir together with a spoon.

6 Season to taste with the sumac and sea salt. Drizzle over a couple of tablespoons of olive oil to taste. It should be enough to just coat the mixture, but not make it too wet. Give the slaw a final stir to mix everything together.

toppers

Perfect with a piece of white fish, such as cod or hake. Add a handful of cooked quinoa for a complete macronutrient-tastic meal.

morph your slaw
Sweet Potato + Lively Lemon Fish Cakes

1 Boil a large, chopped sweet potato until cooked, about 12 minutes. Drain and mash.

2 Mix your slaw into the mash.

3 Add tinned salmon and 1 egg white to bind.

4 Mix together and shape handfuls into patties.

5 Pan-fry or bake at 180°C for 20 minutes.

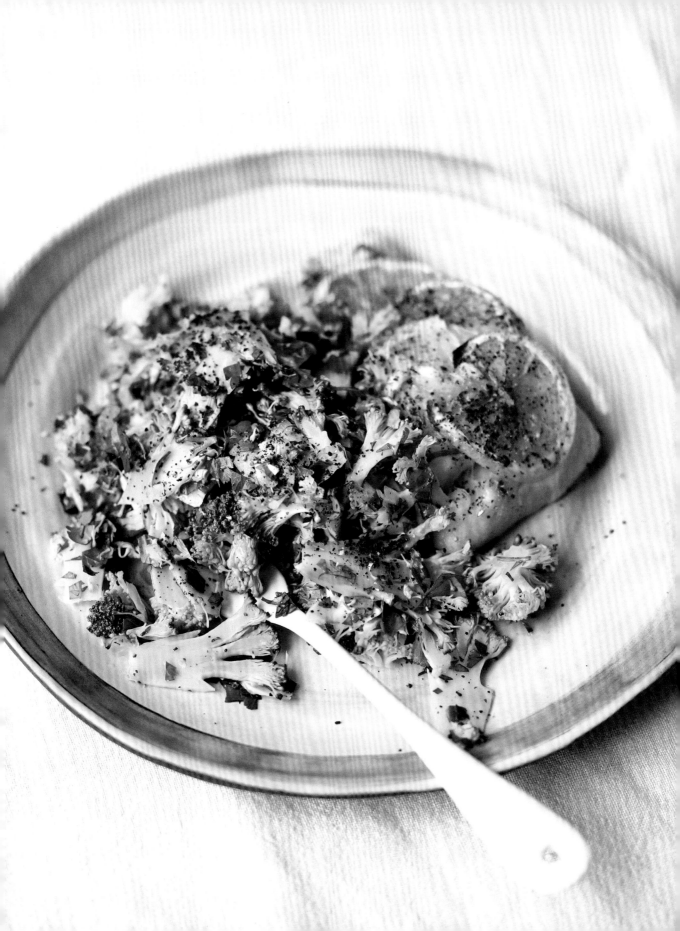

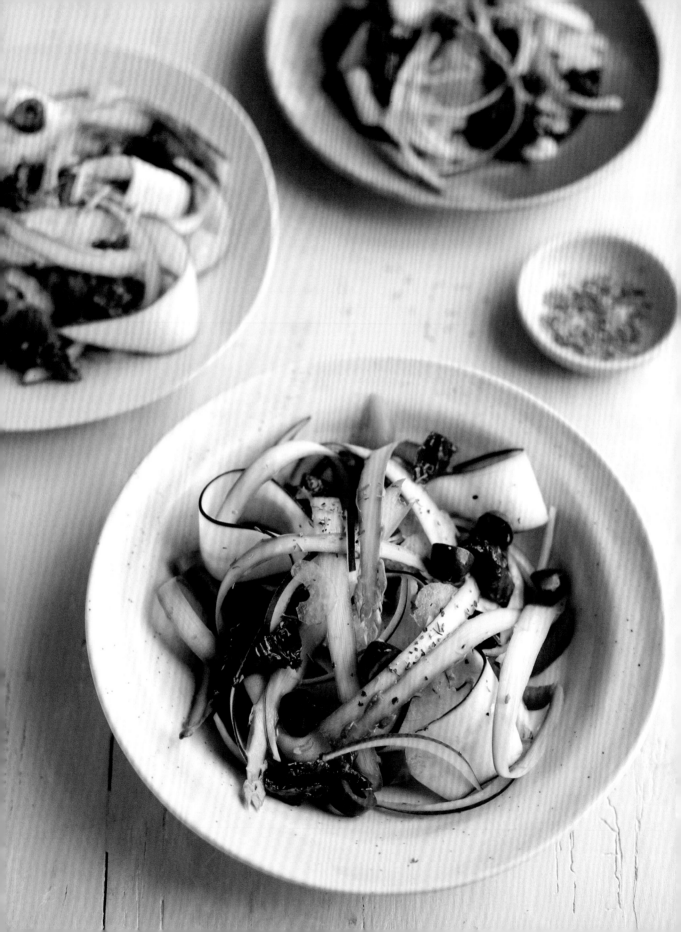

Mediterranean Sunshine Slaw

Sun-dried tomatoes mixed with olives help give any dish a Mediterranean feel. Chopping the olives and tomatoes in the food processor creates a wonderful thick paste to coat the vegetables with but, if you prefer a chunky finish, you can chop these by hand at the end. This recipe has a slightly higher fat content than others in the chapter, so serve with a lean protein like white fish, turkey or chicken. Asparagus can be eaten raw, but you may wish to soften it slightly with a quick blanch.

6–8 spears of asparagus, woody
   ends removed
6–8 stalks of celery, cut into thirds
1 courgette
6–8 sun-dried tomatoes
16 pitted olives
1 red pepper, deseeded
1 green pepper, deseeded
1 small red onion
Drizzle of olive oil
Sprinkle of Mediterranean herbs mix
   (optional)
Sea salt

Makes 4 large portions

1 If blanching the asparagus first, cook for 2 minutes in boiling water, then cool by running under cold water.
2 Place the asparagus along with the celery stalks into the main food processor bowl with the central chopping attachment. Pulse gently until the vegetables are cut into small pieces. Place the mixture into a waiting bowl.
3 Next, add the courgette, sun-dried tomatoes and olives and repeat the 'pulse chop' until chunky. The olives and tomatoes will form a bit of a 'paste' within the mixture. Add to the bowl.
4 Chop the peppers and onion by hand into small cubes. Add to the bowl and mix well.
5 Cover with olive oil and sprinkle with Mediterranean mixed herbs and salt. Mix and serve.

toppers

Top with a prawn and squid seafood mix.

morph your slaw
Baked Mediterranean Vegetable Slaw

1 Take a baking tray and fill with any leftover Mediterranean Sunshine Slaw.
2 Cover with a tin of chopped tomatoes, mix in and bake at 180°C until cooked, about 20 minutes.

Iceberg Tartare Slaw

Iceberg lettuce is a hidden gem for upping hydration through food and pairing some pickles and my creamy protein favourite, quark (see page 127), will prove any iceberg lettuce doubters wrong. This is a tasty staple on days of extra thirst. The dressing in this emulates a tartare sauce, so it's a fabulous pairing to fish. Lettuce is not only hydrating but also provides a fair amount of vitamins A and K, so is super-skin friendly too. Due to its very high water content, be sure not to get carried away in the food processor. This will blitz in seconds!

*1 iceberg lettuce, core removed and
  sliced into large pieces*
2 tablespoons mini cornichons
2 tablespoons drained capers
30 g chives, finely chopped
1 lemon, halved
2–3 tablespoons cider vinegar
2–3 tablespoons olive oil
Sea salt

Makes 4 large portions

1 Place the central chopping attachment into the food processor and add the iceberg lettuce. Pulse very gently until chopped. You may need to do this in batches. Place in a waiting bowl.

2 Add the pickles and chives and repeat the pulsing to form a chunky paste. Pour over the lettuce.

3 Squeeze the lemon juice over the lettuce.

4 Add the vinegar, olive oil and a sprinkle of sea salt to a jam jar. Cover with a lid, shake vigorously and pour over the lettuce mix. Mix everything together well.

toppers

Cooked green peas. You can even pop these into the food processor first and mix with a dash of olive oil and vinegar for a home-made mushy pea TOPPER!

morph your slaw

Tartare Fish + Seafood Salad

1 Flake some pre-cooked white fish into any leftover slaw.

2 Add in a pre-cooked seafood mix.

3 Stir and add a dash of lemon juice and a sprinkle of fresh parsley.

Fresh + Simple Slaw

This was my first ever creation, having got home from work and found these three vegetables sitting alone in my fridge. With few ingredients, it is a 'Super-fast' Slaw to make, and a great alternative to a side salad. Celery is an excellent source of vitamin K and supplies vitamins A and C, serving as a crunchy but hydrating low-calorie base for any slaw. Make in large batches and use throughout the week.

1 head (400 g) of broccoli, cut into
  quarters
1 bag (150 g) of sugar snap peas
10 stalks of celery
2 limes, halved
Drizzle of olive oil
Sea salt

Makes 4 large portions

1 Place the central chopping attachment into the main bowl of the food processor.

2 Place the broccoli in the bowl and replace the lid. Pulse it, in short bursts, into finer pieces. Be careful not to over-pulse – you want the broccoli to remain coarse and chunky, not powdery. Tip the broccoli into a waiting bowl.

3 Repeat the above with the sugar snap peas, pulsing briefly until chopped (this will take seconds).

4 Remove the blade and add the flat 'chopper' blade on to the top. Replace the lid. Place the celery into the opening at the top while turning the food processor on. Push it through with the added attachment until sliced. Add to the bowl.

5 Squeeze the juice of the 2 limes and a drizzle of olive oil over the mix.

6 Sprinkle with sea salt and mix well.

toppers

Dehydrated kale chips.

morph your slaw

Fresh + Simple Tuna Salad Twist

1 Mash an avocado.

2 Mix with a tin of no drain tuna.

3 Add in any leftover slaw and mix well.

Ruby Green Slaw

Pomegranate seeds add a lovely jewelled sparkle of ruby red and are well known for their high levels of antioxidants, which makes the little bit of work trying to get them out of the skin worthwhile!

If using whole pomegranates, here is a tip (courtesy of Jamie Oliver). Place the pomegranate into the freezer for a few minutes, then remove, place onto its side and slice in half. Slightly squeeze, then turn upside down above a large bowl. With a strong motion, tap the bottom repeatedly with a wooden spoon and the seeds will fall out. Remove any pith.

1 head (large size) of Chinese leaf, core removed and sliced into sixteenths
3 heads of pak choi, cores removed
2 small heads of chicory, sliced into sixths
2 green chillies, deseeded
3 large handfuls of coriander
Juice of 1 small orange
2–3 tablespoons olive oil
Himalayan pink sea salt (or rock salt or standard sea salt)
1 pomegranate, deseeded or 2 packets (100 g) of pomegranate seeds

Makes 4 large portions

1 Place the central chopping attachment into the main bowl of the food processor, followed by the Chinese leaf and pak choi. Pulse gently until a chunky chop, then tip into a waiting bowl.
2 Next, add the chicory heads, chillies and coriander. Repeat until chopped. Add to the bowl.
3 Cover the vegetables with the orange juice and olive oil.
4 Add the sea salt and mix well.
5 Sprinkle with the pomegranate seeds.

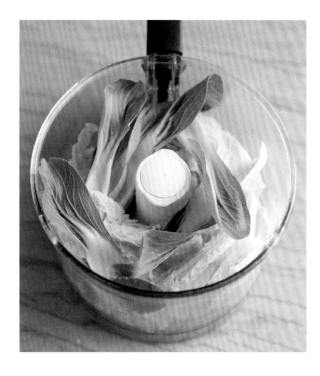

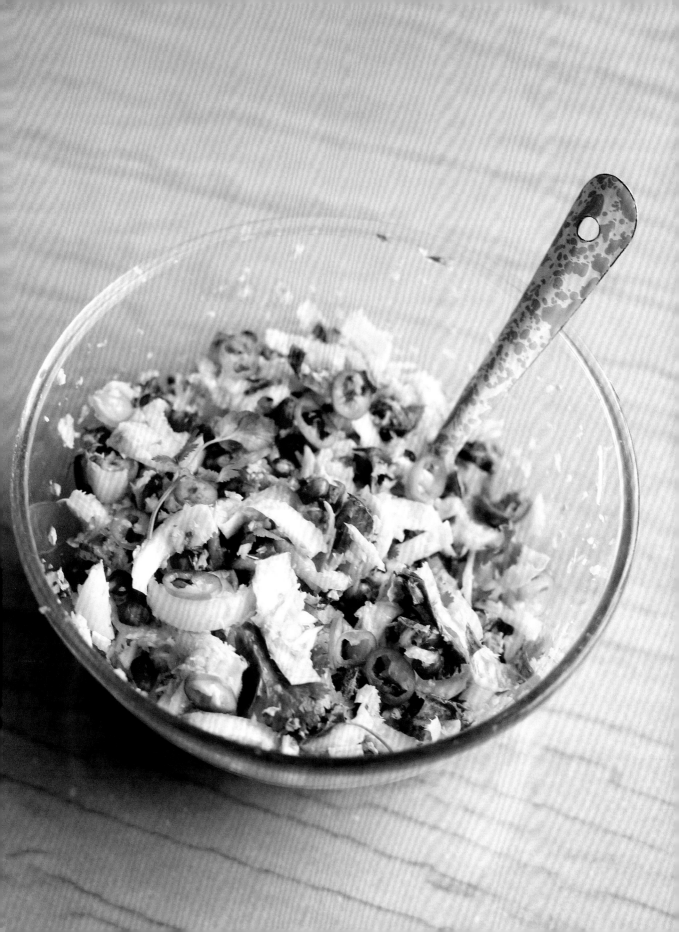

toppers

The sweet-and-sour pomegranate flavour works really well when served with fruit. For an extra vitamin C kick, top with some clementine or orange segments for a 'veggie' fruity salad. Add parsley leaves to serve.

morph your slaw
Ruby Green Cheese Slaw

1 Slice a goat's cheese log and place the cheese onto baking paper under a medium grill.
2 Grill until melted or golden brown.
3 Place the cheese on top of the slaw and let it melt into the leaves.

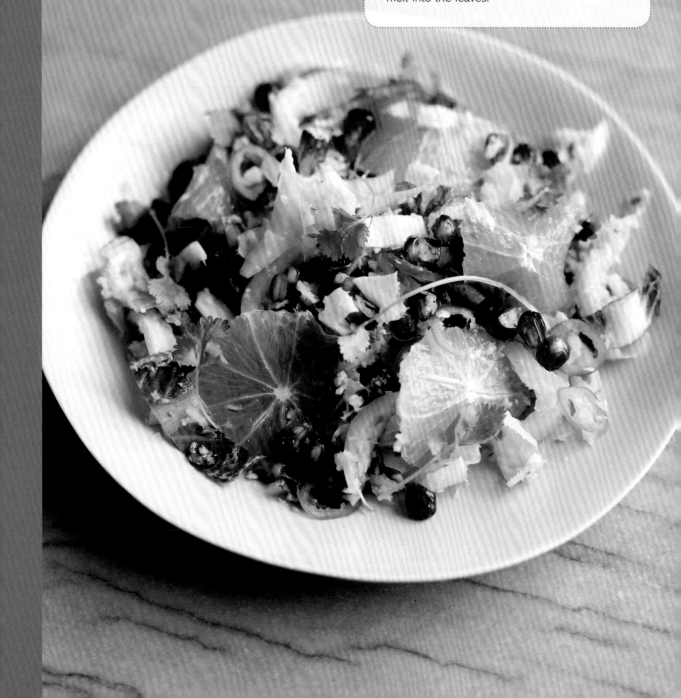

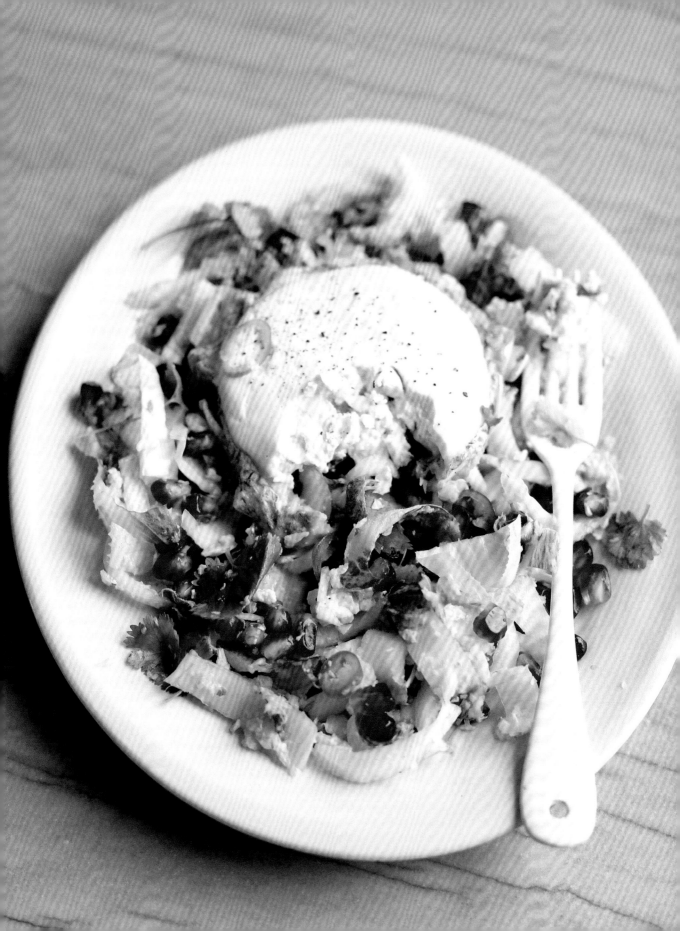

Fresh + Minty Slaw

I really love raw green beans, however some people (namely my other half!) like to have theirs slightly blanched to bring out the flavour. So in the interests of keeping a happy man at home... I do occasionally pour some boiling water in a bowl and leave the beans to slightly blanch for a few minutes before I chop them. Experiment with both and see which you prefer.

Mint is a known as a calming and soothing herb, helping digestive problems if you've had a weekend of food indulgence! This is a super-fresh and very light slaw, so it can be used alone as a bit of a palate or digestive cleanser. Conversely, it can really help balance a dense, heavier meal or meat, so works well with lamb or beef.

1 bag (150 g) of mixed green beans
8–10 stalks of celery
1 large handful of flat-leaf parsley
1 large handful of mint
2–3 tablespoons olive oil
2–3 tablespoons white wine vinegar
Sea salt
1–2 teaspoons dried mint (optional)

Makes 4 large portions

MORPH pictured

1 Place your (either blanched or raw) green beans and celery into the main bowl of the food processor. Pulse gently until you have small chunky-chopped pieces. Remove and add to a waiting bowl.

2 Next, add your herbs (alternatively you can hand-chop). Herbs will mush into a paste easily in a food processor, so they will then coat the vegetables well with their flavour.

3 Add the herbs to the chopped vegetables.

4 Add the olive oil, vinegar and a sprinkle of sea salt to a jam jar. Place the lid on and shake vigorously. Pour over the slaw.

5 Sprinkle with the dried mint and mix well.

toppers

Watermelon works really well with minty flavours as both are fresh and hydrating. Top this slaw with cubes of melon to serve as a light summer-drenched bite.

morph your slaw
Mediterranean Lamb Chop SuperSlaw

1 Sprinkle some Mediterranean herbs over two lamb chops.

2 Pan-fry or grill lamb chops in a little oil until cooked, about 4 minutes on each side.

3 Serve topped on leftover slaw.

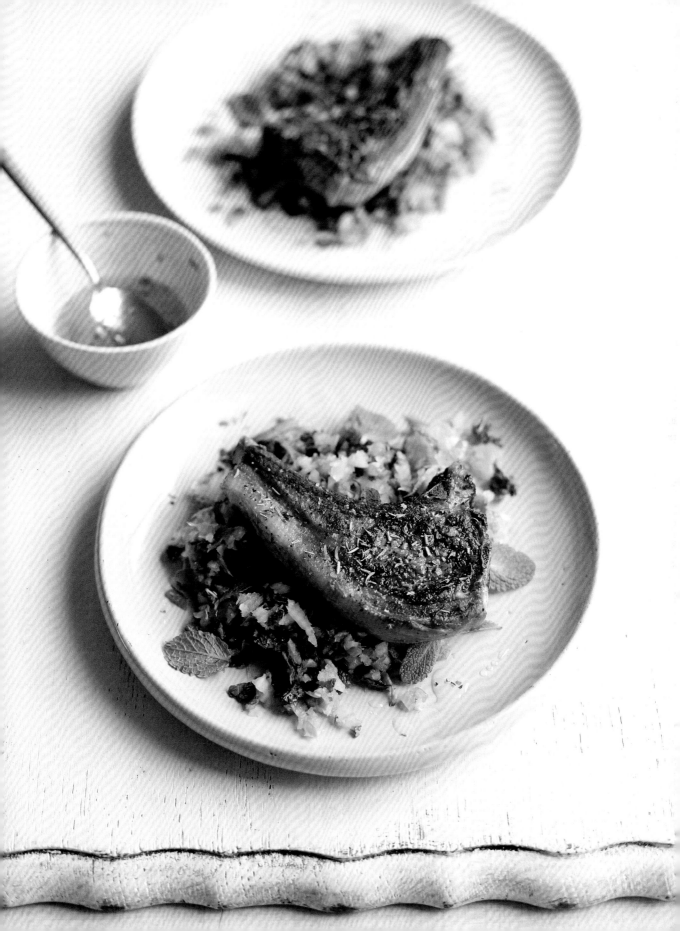

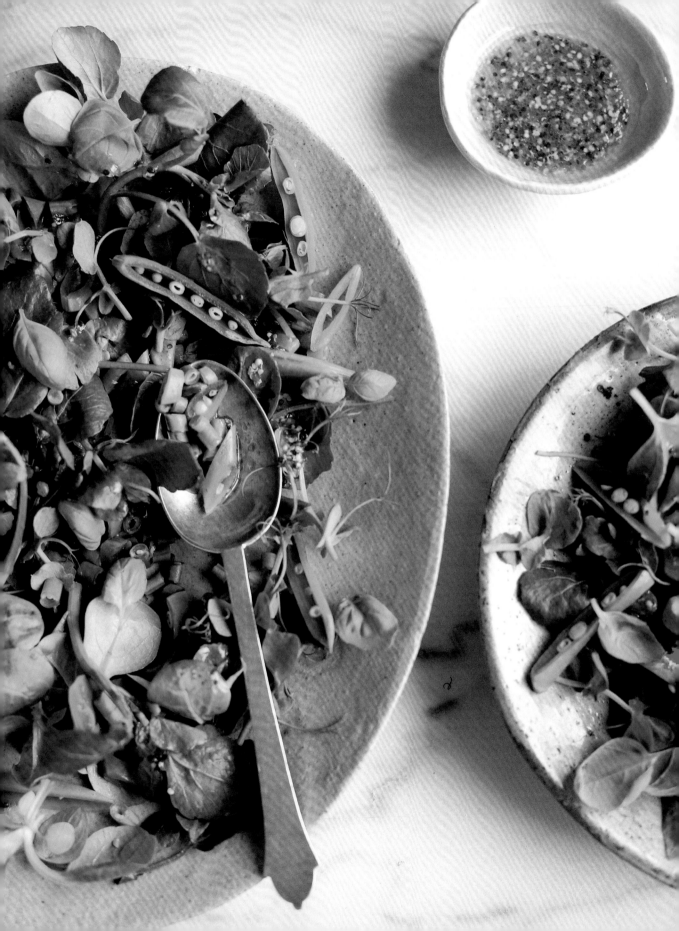

Watercress, Beans + Basil Slaw

Fresh, good-quality mixed leaves can really make a slaw. If you lack time to visit a local greengrocers, lamb's lettuce and pea shoots can be found pre-mixed and bagged in most supermarkets. Make sure you check the base of the bag to see the condition of the leaf. If they aren't fresh you'll notice a build up of green sludge at the bottom. Spinach and rocket make a great alternative. Fresh leaves don't last long when dressed, so this slaw is best eaten fresh.

1 bag (150 g) of green beans
1 bag (150 g) of mangetout
1 handful of basil leaves
2–3 handfuls of mixed leaves or lamb's lettuce and mixed pea shoots
2–3 large handfuls of watercress
3–4 tablespoons olive oil
1 heaped tablespoon wholegrain mustard
2–3 tablespoons cider vinegar
Himalayan pink sea salt

Makes 4 large portions

1 Place the central chopping attachment into the main bowl of the food processor and add the green beans (either steamed or raw) and mangetout. Pulse until chopped into chunky pieces. Place in a waiting bowl.

2 Place the basil, mixed leaves and watercress into the bowl and repeat. This will take seconds to pulse into a finer chop. Mix in with the vegetables.

3 Add the olive oil, mustard and vinegar to a jam jar. Place the lid on and shake vigorously. Pour over the slaw.

4 Season with sea salt and mix well.

toppers

Watercress can handle strong or smoky flavours. Top with some chopped pieces of smoked salmon or mackerel.

morph your slaw
Creamy Watercress Mustard Slaw

1 Mix in a blob or two of Greek or natural yoghurt to the slaw for a creamier and more subtle-flavoured SuperSlaw.

Za'atar Slaw

I found the za'atar herb mix in a local deli – however I've seen it in many places since (even Oxfam!) It's a pre-made aromatic herb mix, which is delicious – it's basically made from olive oil, sea salt, thyme and sumac. If you can't find it or don't already have it in stock, just replace this with your own mix of sea salt, sumac and dried thyme.

1 large Chinese leaf cabbage, core removed and sliced into thirds
½ head (75 g) of broccoli
1 bag (200 g) of mixed green cabbage leaves (for ease you can buy these pre-shredded in packets at most local supermarkets)
3–4 tablespoons olive oil
1 teaspoon Dijon mustard
2 lemons, halved
Za'atar herb mix
Sea salt

Makes 4 large portions

TOPPER pictured

1 Place the central chopping attachment into the main bowl of the food processor and add the Chinese leaf. Pulse for seconds until a chunky chop is achieved. Add to a waiting bowl.

2 Add the broccoli and repeat, chopping until a chunky consistency.

3 Repeat with the mixed cabbage greens. If they are already very finely chopped when you buy them, then you can add straight in without chopping if you wish.

4 Add the olive oil and mustard to a jam jar. Place the lid on and shake vigorously. Pour over the slaw.

5 Squeeze with fresh lemon juice.

6 Sprinkle with the za'atar and sea salt and mix well.

toppers

Nut lover? All nuts make a great crunchy topper for this slaw, although the tangy tone of walnuts pairs well with za'atar's lemony flavours.

morph your slaw

Honey + Sesame Za'atar Chicken

1 In a pan over a medium heat, cook strips of chicken in a little sesame oil until done, about 8 minutes.

2 Add any leftover slaw to the pan and fry for 1–2 minutes.

3 Drizzle with a teaspoon of honey and mix well.

4 Serve with a sprinkle of sesame seeds and some pre-cooked basmati rice.

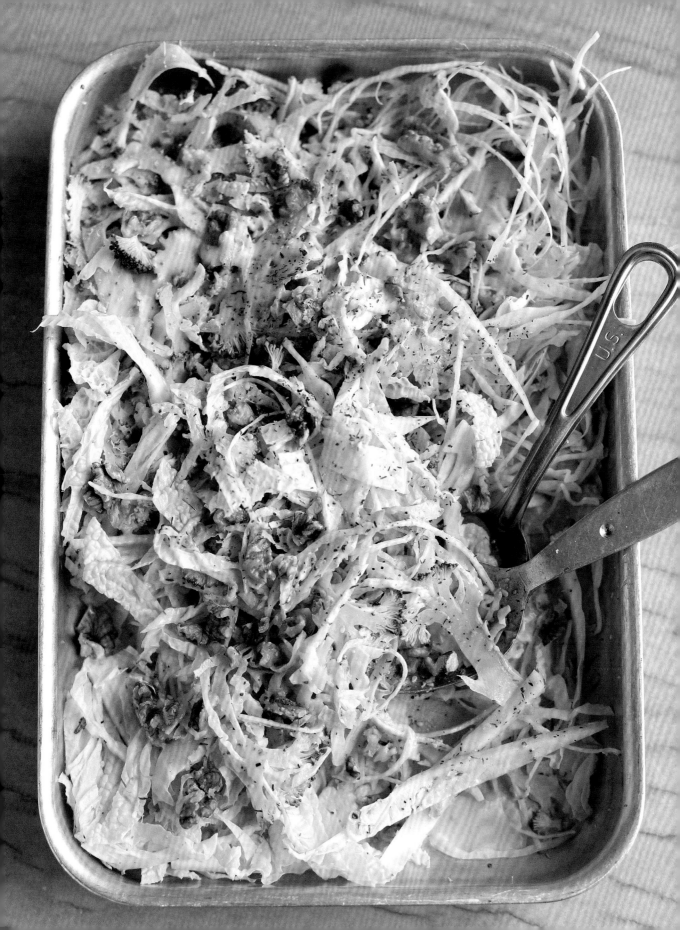

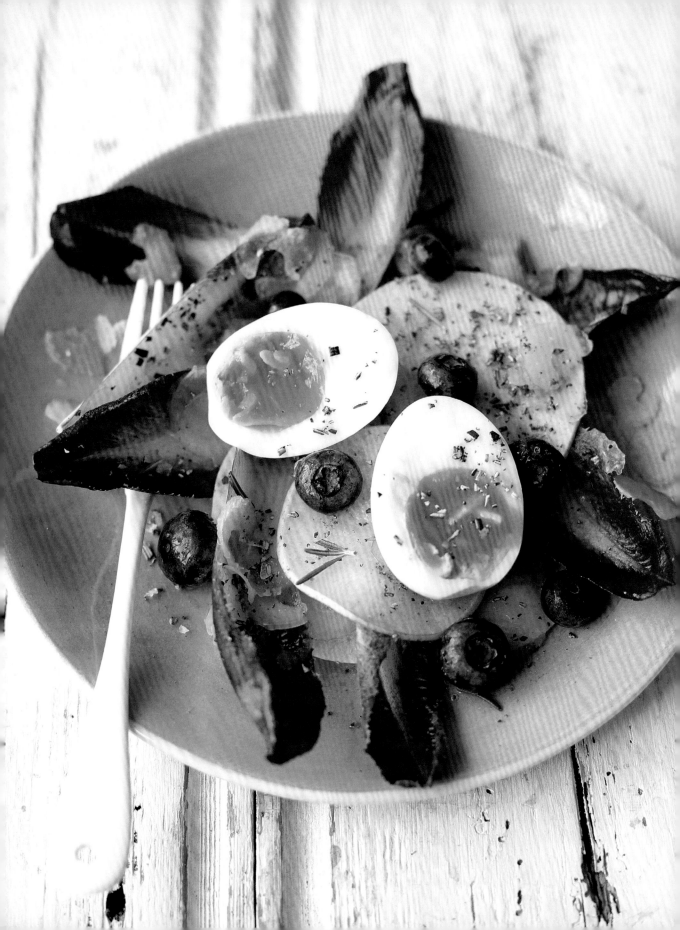

Chicory Pear Slaw

Try and go for firmer pears, as generally they stay fresher in the slaw for longer (leave any softer fruits for the end). If you can source them, Asian pears work really well and look like a large golden apple – a thirst-quenching snack, I became addicted when I visited the wet markets of Hong Kong. The morph for this Slaw may sound bizarre, but trust me; it works, is delicious and has become an absolute staple in my meal plans.

2 firm green or Asian pears,
  cores removed
1 small head of red chicory,
  quartered
8–10 stalks of celery
1 tablespoon chopped rosemary
2 lemons, halved and deseeded
2–3 tablespoons olive oil
Celery salt
Sea salt

Makes 4 large portions

MORPH pictured

1 Place the central chopping attachment into the food processor and add the pears and the chicory. Pulse gently until chopped into chunky pieces. Place in a waiting bowl.
2 Repeat, adding in the celery and rosemary. Chop for seconds and add to the bowl.
3 Squeeze the juice of the lemons over the mix.
4 Drizzle with olive oil and sprinkle with celery salt and sea salt. Mix well.

toppers

Apparently the king of the anti-ageing fruits, a handful of blueberries will top this slaw beautifully!

morph your slaw

Frozen Blueberry + Egg Salad

1 Boil or poach an egg per person, until the eggs are just runny. If poaching this will take about 3 minutes, boiling will take 5 minutes.
2 Plate any leftover Chicory Pear and sprinkle over a handful of frozen blueberries.
3 Slice the eggs in half and place on top of the plate of Slaw.
4 Season to taste with sea salt and pepper and serve.

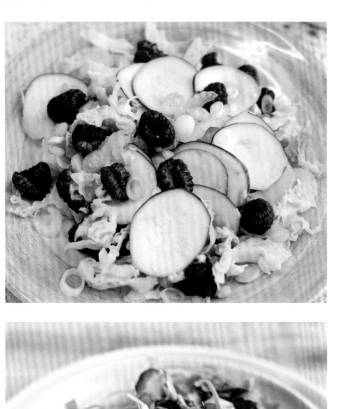

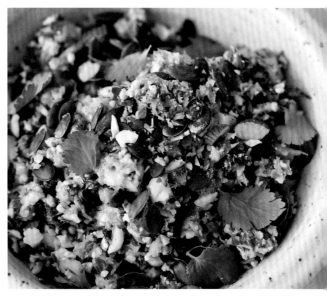

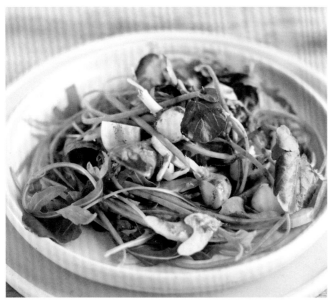

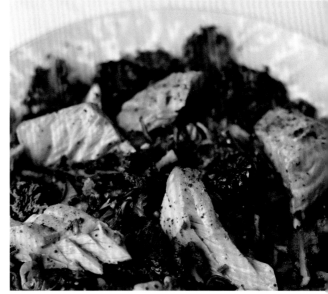

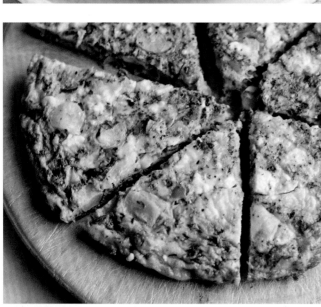

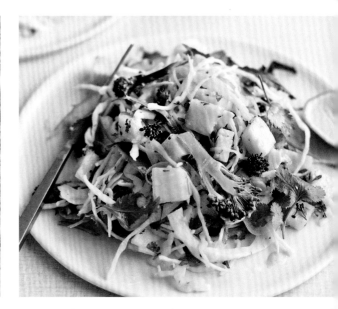

Immunity

Our immune system helps in our defence against illness and disease. As with all things health based, there is a huge amount about the immune system and how it functions that we still don't understand. What we do know, however, is that the way to maintain it is to strive for balance in all areas, including nutrition. Working hard, playing hard and managing busy routines, often with less sleep than we would like, all place stress on our bodies and minds. Over time, the balance can tip and we can find ourselves feeling run down.

Learning when to slow down in life is something we should probably all work on. When I feel the start of a cold, the first thing I do is plan a rest day, even if this just means allotting time for an extra hour of snooze! Sleep helps us recover. Rest helps us switch off a racing mind, both of which play a role in helping your immune system fight illness. While we rest, the body needs a plethora of vitamins and minerals. Research indicates that various micronutrient deficiencies alter immune responses, making the body more susceptible to illness.

So, combine a good old rest day with a vitamin-loaded SuperSlaw. These recipes and recommended TOPPERS contain ingredients high in vitamin C, zinc and have anti-inflammatory benefits to help your immune system do its work.

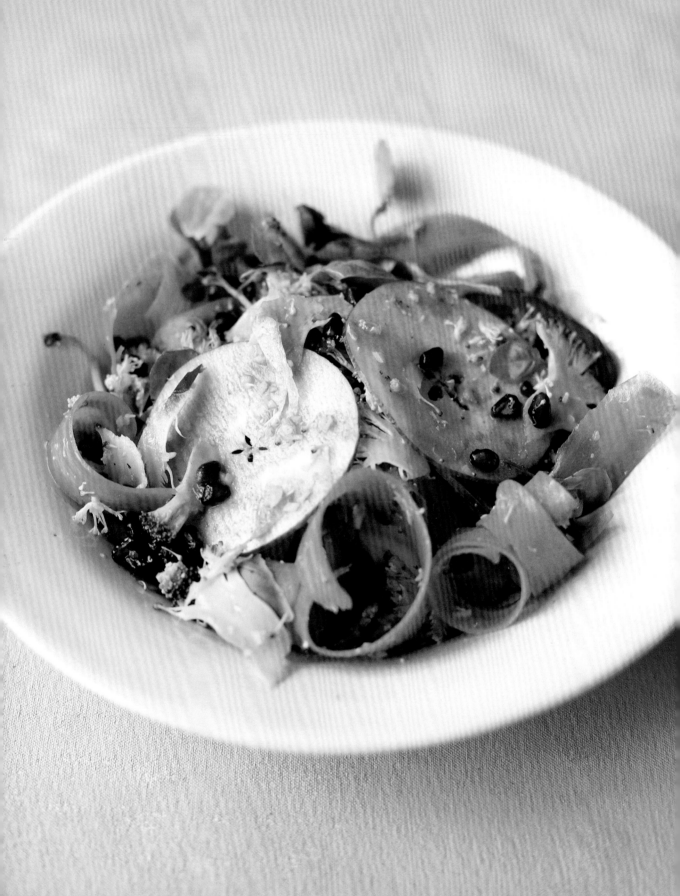

Vit-Kick Slaw

My go-to spices when I feel unwell are turmeric and ginger. Known to contain heaps of anti-inflammatory benefits, they are also really easy to source and add into many dishes. This dish is a powerhouse of vitamins, reflected in the rainbow of colour. I often challenge my clients to make one dietary change a week. One of the easiest goals I set them is increasing their use of natural colour in the foods that they prepare. Science shows adults are more likely to eat healthful foods if there are more than three colours on the plate (for children it's six), so test yourself and see how much rainbow food you can serve to your family. There is a reason why synthetic food colourings exist – an important part of how we eat is visual. Carrots and pomegranates provide sweetness, heaps of vitamins and antioxidants, making them natural SuperSlaw supplements.

6–8 carrots, peeled
½ head (200 g) of broccoli
2–3 large handfuls of watercress
1 apple (I use Pink Lady as they
    are big and extra sweet, but feel
    free to swap in your personal
    favourite), core removed and
    peeled
1 small cube of fresh ginger, peeled
½ teaspoon ground turmeric
1 lemon, halved and deseeded
1 red pepper, deseeded
½ pomegranate, deseeded (see
    page 30) or 1 packet (50 g) of
    pomegranate seeds
3–4 tablespoons olive oil
Sea salt

Makes 4 large portions

TOPPER pictured

1 Place the central chopping attachment into the main bowl of the food processor and add in the carrots. Pulse until chopped. Carrots are dense vegetables so don't worry about the noise, just aim for a consistency of slice. Tip into a waiting bowl.

2 Add the broccoli and watercress to the food processor bowl and repeat. Add to the chopped carrot and mix well.

3 Now add the apple and ginger and again pulse until finely chopped, making sure the ginger hasn't been missed (you can chop the ginger finely by hand if you want to ensure a fine slice).

4 Tip all of the vegetables together and stir in the turmeric. Squeeze over the lemon juice and mix.

5 Hand-slice the pepper and stir into the mix. Finally, add in the pomegranate seeds and stir well.

6 Drizzle with the olive oil and a sprinkle of sea salt and mix.

toppers

Basil is a lovely fragrant herb that gives an extra antibacterial top for this slaw; just add a roughly torn handful before serving.

morph your slaw

Ham Asparagus Vit-Kick Rolls

1 Lightly steam a handful of asparagus spears for about 5 minutes.

2 Lay out slices of Parma ham and spoon any leftover slaw down the middle of the sheets.

3 Add an asparagus spear to the top of each slice and roll the ham around the slaw to cover.

4 Place each parcel under a medium grill. Turn frequently and cook until lightly browned.

5 Finish by lightly grating over a little Parmesan.

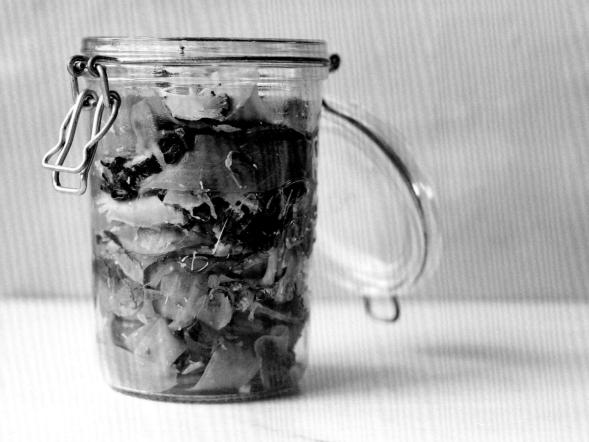

Iron Maiden Slaw

Many lifestyle factors can lead to a depletion of iron levels, and women and those who train for endurance exercise are identified as being more at risk of this common cause of fatigue. Keep your iron levels boosted naturally with dark green leafy vegetables, such as kale and spinach. TOPPERS high in vitamin C help the body to absorb non-heme iron (the type found in vegetable sources), so chop up some tomatoes or kiwi to maximize the benefits.

200 g kale
1 large bag (200 g) of spinach
3 handfuls of watercress
1 handful of basil
1 red onion, thinly sliced by hand
3–4 tablespoons olive oil
2–3 tablespoons balsamic vinegar
Sea salt and freshly ground black
* pepper*

Makes 4 large portions

1 Place the central chopping attachment into the main bowl in the food processor and add in the kale. Pulse gently until chopped into small pieces. Add to a waiting bowl.
2 Next, add the spinach, watercress and basil. Repeat the pulse motion until finely chopped.
3 Mix the ingredients together, adding in the hand-sliced onion (you can add into the food processor if you wish, just keep your eye on how fine it chops).
4 Mix the olive oil and balsamic in a jam jar. Replace the lid and shake vigorously. Pour over the mixture.
5 Season with sea salt and pepper and mix well.

toppers
Chopped cherry tomatoes and slices of kiwi.

morph your slaw
Iron Maiden Hot Salsa

1 Fry some sliced red chilli and a tin of chopped tomatoes over a medium heat for 5 minutes.
2 Add in any leftover slaw and heat through for a further few minutes.

Crunchy slaw

There is a lot of love for horseradish as a natural way to clear congestion from cold and flu symptoms. Almonds are high in zinc and a great source of heart-healthy, mono-unsaturated fat. Horseradish mustard can be bought, but you can make your own by mixing ½ teaspoon Dijon mustard with ½ teaspoon horseradish sauce if you don't have this to hand.

1 head (400 g) of broccoli, cut into
    quarters
200 g kale
6–8 stalks of celery, cut into thirds
1 courgette, cut into thirds
1 bag (150 g) of sugar snap peas
2 handfuls of coriander
2 handfuls of skin-on almonds
1 green chilli, deseeded
1 tablespoon horseradish mustard
4 tablespoons olive oil
4 tablespoons white wine vinegar
1 teaspoon Dijon mustard
Sea salt
2 handfuls of pumpkin seeds
Coriander leaves, to garnish

Makes 4 large portions

1 Place the central chopping attachment into the main bowl of the food processor.

2 Place the broccoli in the bowl, then add the kale and replace the lid. Blend with the pulse button until chunky, then add to a waiting bowl. You may need to do this in stages.

3 Add the celery and courgette to the food processor along with the sugar snap peas. Pulse to a chunky-chopped texture and stir into the broccoli and kale mix.

4 Roughly hand-chop the coriander and mix with the vegetables.

5 Place the almonds and chilli into the bottom of the food processor and whizz for a brief second to chop. You could also chop the chilli by hand and crush the almonds with a pestle and mortar, if you prefer. Add to the vegetables and mix.

6 Add the horseradish, olive oil, vinegar, mustard and a sprinkle of sea salt to an empty jam jar. Put the lid on tight and shake vigorously until mixed. Pour the dressing over the slaw.

7 Mix well and garnish with the pumpkin seeds and some coriander.

toppers

Strong flavours complement this slaw's fabulously fiery taste. Try topping with grilled tomatoes and a few slices of grilled lean bacon.

morph your slaw
Hot Steak Salad

1 Pan-fry mushrooms and onions for 15 minutes over a low heat.

2 Fry a steak for 7 minutes, turning every minute.

3 Add your slaw and mushroom mix to the steak pan and heat for a couple of minutes.

4 Serve as a hot steak salad.

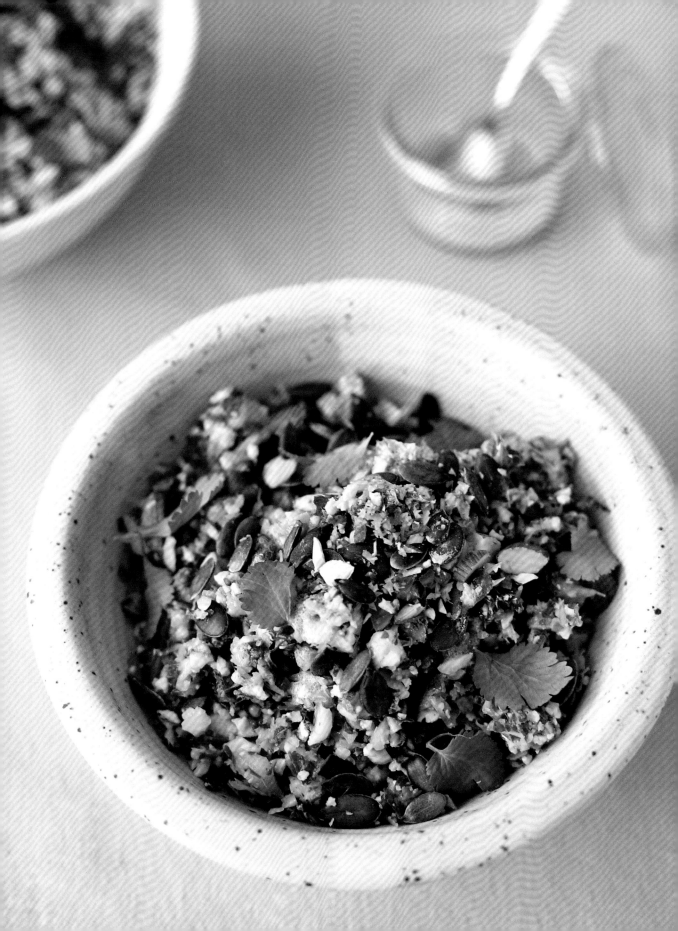

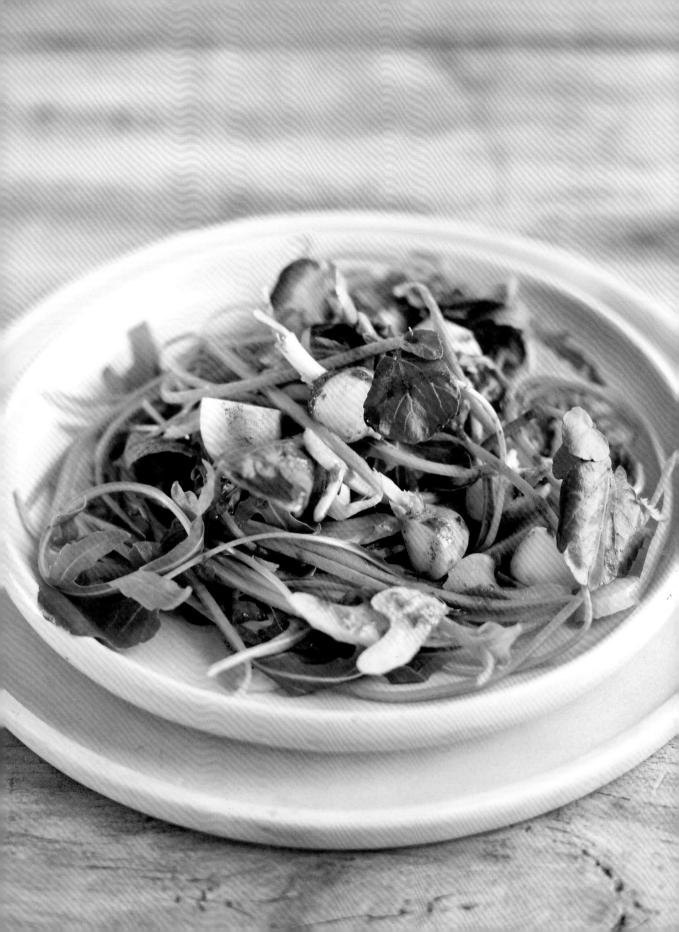

Baby Turnip Fire Slaw

Sweet paprika helps to provide a red, fiery coating to the baby turnips, which gives a beautiful appearance. Baby turnips have long been used in Chinese medicine as a decongestant, although they are often overlooked for their larger counterparts. Try and track them down in the root vegetable section of your supermarket. Turnips are a good source of vitamin C and you can make great use of the turnip greens to top your slaw – rich in vitamins A and E the greens are also super-rich in calcium.

4 baby turnips, peeled and cores removed (don't forget to keep the greens!)
6 stalks of celery
4 carrots, peeled
3 large handfuls of mixed rocket, spinach and watercress (I used a pre-mixed bag for this)
1½ lemons
1 teaspoon sweet paprika
3–4 tablespoons olive oil
Sea salt

Makes 4 large portions

1 Place the central chopping attachment into the main bowl of the food processor.
2 Place the turnips into the bowl and replace the lid. Pulse until thickly chopped. Turnips are hard root vegetables, so they will be noisy. Hold your hand down firmly on the top. Add to a waiting bowl.
3 Add the celery and repeat the pulse process until chopped. Add to the turnips.
4 Repeat with the carrots and mixed leaves. Add to the bowl and mix.
5 Squeeze the lemons over the mix, then add the paprika.
6 Drizzle with olive oil until coated. Mix well. Season with sea salt.

morph your slaw

Baby Turnip Fire + Tofu Stir-Fry

1 Pan-fry chopped garlic cloves in oil for 2 minutes.
2 Add in a handful of green olives.
3 Add in any leftover slaw and heat through.
4 Add in 1 tomato, chopped into cubes, and continue to fry for 1–2 minutes.
5 Stir in some slices of tofu and cook for 5 minutes.
6 Serve with cooked mixed grains or as a simple bowl of stir-fry.

toppers

Sprinkle with chopped turnip greens for an extra calcium kick!

Go-Go Greens

Go-Go Greenwood was a name once given to me by my weightlifting trainer, so I thought it appropriate to create a slaw with heaps of strong green colours in his honour! Japanese mustard spinach (komatsuna) is similar to (standard) spinach with a slightly less bitter taste. If you can't find this easily, just add in a little extra spinach or even a few handfuls of kale. Go-Go Greens provides an awesome green base for most meals. This is the type of slaw that MORPHS well into many other dishes.

150 g spinach
1 large handful of basil
200 g Japanese mustard spinach
   (if you cannot source this, then
   you can increase the amount of
   standard spinach instead)
1 bag (150 g) of sugar snap peas
12 stalks of celery
12 radishes, topped and tailed
16 small green olives
1 tablespoon cider vinegar
1 tablespoon balsamic vinegar
3–4 tablespoons olive oil
Himalayan pink sea salt

Makes 4 large portions

1 Place the central chopping attachment into the main bowl of the food processor and add in the spinach, basil and mustard spinach. Pulse until chopped. This will take seconds and will quickly become very fine. Tip into a waiting bowl.

2 Add the sugar snap peas and celery into the food processor and repeat until chopped more coarsely. Add to the mix.

3 You can chop the radishes and olives by hand into very small pieces or add to the food processor to chop, then mix in with the other vegetables.

4 Place the vinegars, olive oil and sea salt into a jam jar. Place the lid on and shake vigorously. Pour over the slaw and mix well.

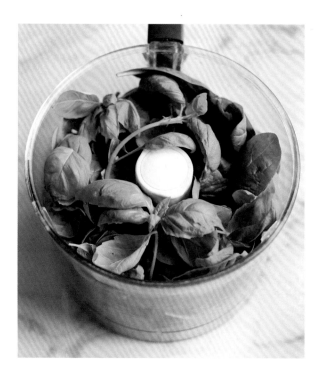

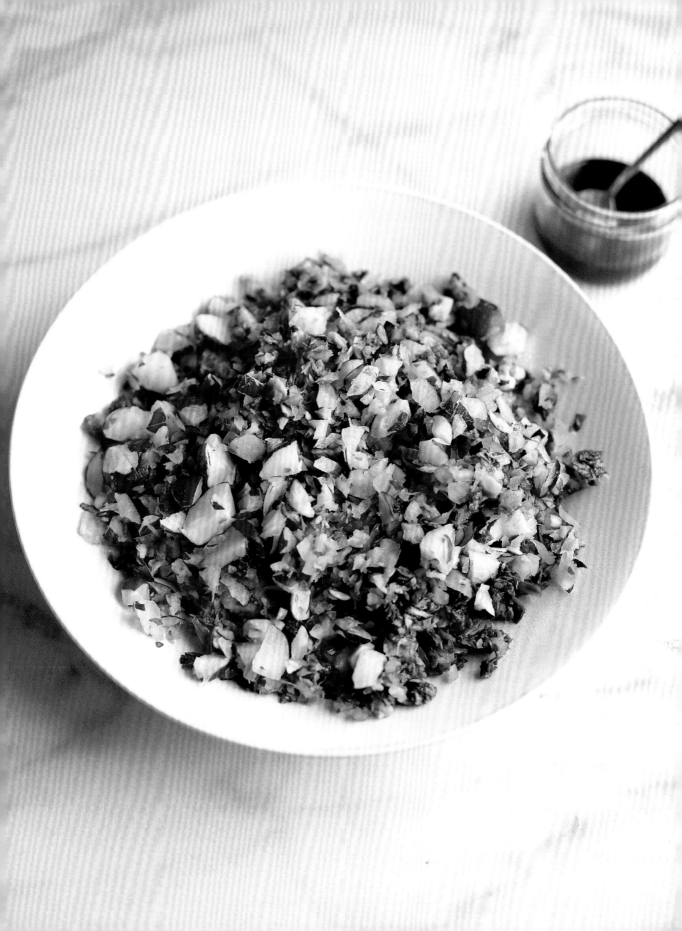

toppers

Add a crumble of feta cheese.

morph your slaw
Green Greek Omelette

1 Take any leftover slaw and add to a bowl with 3 eggs. Whisk until mixed.
2 Crumble in some feta cheese.
3 Fry in a shallow-based pan in a little oil until cooked through. Place under a medium grill for a few minutes until golden brown.

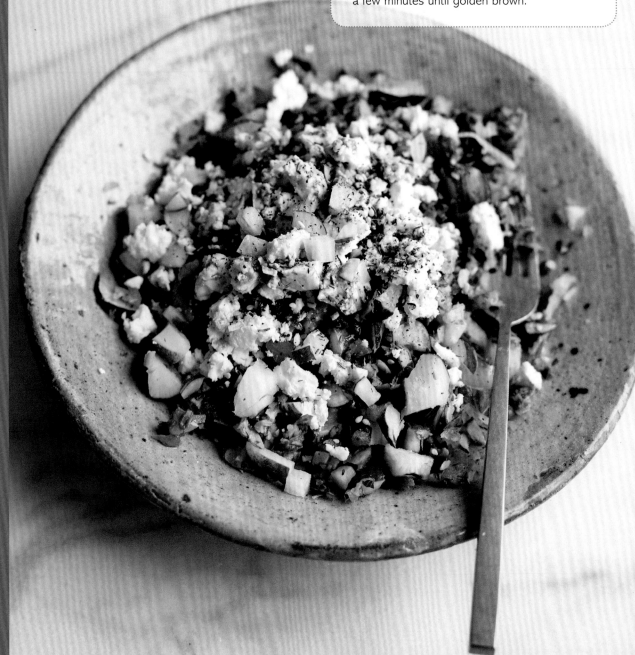

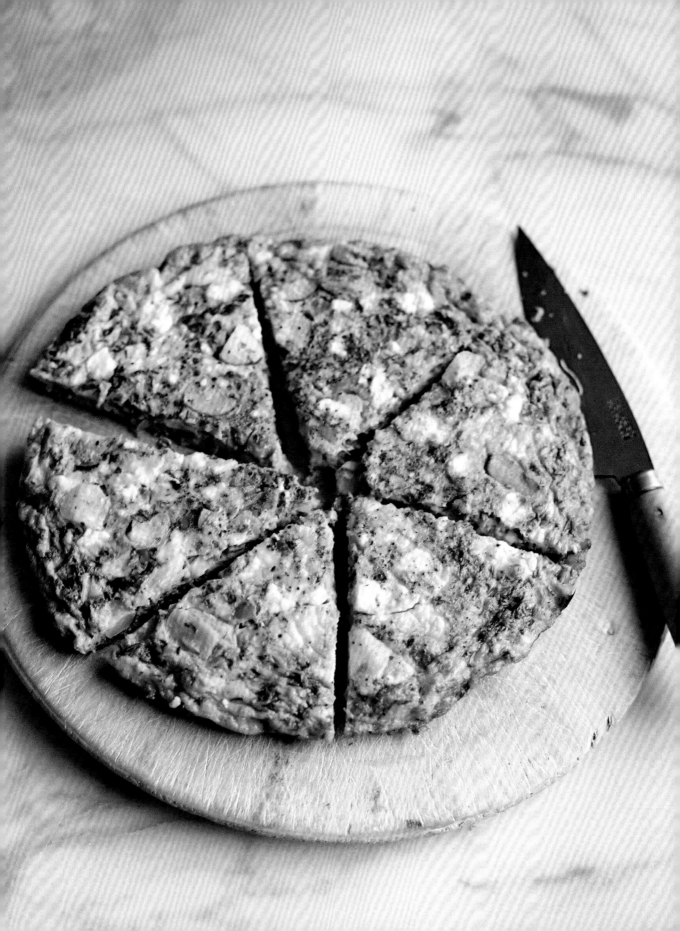

Sweet Onion Slaw

In terms of immune system health, raw onions seem to pack a powerful punch against cold and flu symptoms. A good friend used to swear by raw onion consumption as his own self-medication whenever he felt rundown. Maybe not the ideal food for a first date, but with natural antibacterial agents, onions can help the body deal with unwanted viruses. Quercetin is a plant compound found in onions, which is said to be strongly linked with boosting a healthy immunity. With natural anti-histamine properties it can help lessen the effects of hayfever. Eat soon after production.

1 large red onion
½ small white or green cabbage,
  core removed
1 bag (150 g) of sugar snap peas
1 heaped teaspoon Dijon mustard
3–4 tablespoons olive oil
½ teaspoon cranberry sauce
Sea salt

Makes 4 large portions

1 Place the central chopping attachment into the main bowl of the food processor and add the onion. Pulse until finely chopped and tip into a waiting bowl.

2 Add the cabbage and sugar snap peas into the food processor and repeat to create a chunky chop. Mix into the onion.

3 Pour the mustard, olive oil, cranberry sauce and a sprinkle of sea salt into an empty jam jar. Place the lid on and shake vigorously. If the cranberry sauce is particularly thick, you will have to keep shaking and checking the jar to make sure it is mixed in. If you need to thin the dressing, add a little more vinegar.

4 Pour over the slaw and mix well.

toppers

Wilted spinach gives this slaw an extra boost of immune-friendly beta-carotene (vitamin A).

morph your slaw
Baked Sweet Onion Trout

1 Line a baking dish with any leftover slaw.

2 Pour over ½ tin of chopped tomatoes.

3 Place a piece of trout on top and bake at 180°C until cooked through, about 20 minutes.

Allotment Slaw

This slaw was made after a kind donation of wonderfully fresh herbs gifted from a beautiful fellow gym bunny Mahnaz, after her allotment had blossomed and she was overrun with produce. Using homegrown, seasonal foods will always make your slaw taste extra special. Wild garlic is reported to help cleanse and support the immune system. It has a very pungent flavour when eaten raw, balanced well with a little fruitiness from the apple. I chop this slaw by hand due to the texture of some of the leaves.

3 handfuls of Swiss chard, roughly chopped
2–3 handfuls of flat-leaf parsley, roughly chopped
3–4 tablespoons drained capers
150 g spinach leaves, roughly chopped
1 small handful of wild garlic, roughly chopped
2 green apples (I use Granny Smith, but feel free to swap), cores removed and chopped
Drizzle of cider vinegar
Drizzle of olive oil
Sea salt

Makes 4 large portions

1 Mix together the Swiss chard and parsley into a waiting bowl.
2 Stir in the drained capers (you may want to rinse them a little to dilute the briny flavour).
3 Add the spinach leaves and wild garlic into the mix.
4 Add in the cored and chopped apple.
5 Add enough vinegar and olive oil to a jam jar to lightly coat the leaves. Add a sprinkle of sea salt. Place the lid on and shake vigorously.
6 Pour over the slaw and mix together well.

toppers

Creamy TOPPERS ease the strong flavours of this slaw. If you tolerate dairy well, try a scoop of natural or Greek yoghurt, quark or crème fraîche.

morph your slaw

Creamy Allotment Quick Pan-fry

1 Add any leftover Allotment Slaw into a pan with some sliced mushrooms and onions and pan fry for about 10 minutes.
2 Add a dash of cream.
3 Serve as a side or as a main with a piece of fish.

Purple Power Slaw

Purple is a bit of a power colour in nature. Studies reveal that purple foods tend to be higher in anthocyanin, a powerful antioxidant. Most supermarkets have got into the purple groove with many unusual new purple vegetable varieties becoming standard on their shelves. It is a great way of getting more colours into your diet and an easy way to make your dishes look more exciting and sneak in those extra vitamins.

1 small or ½ larger red cabbage, core removed and chopped into large chunks
150 g purple sprouting broccoli
100 g purple kale sprouts
1 small handful of green beans, topped and tailed
1 small handful of purple mangetout
2–3 tablespoons balsamic vinegar
3–4 tablespoons olive oil
Sea salt
Sumac

Makes 4 large portions

TOPPER pictured

1 Place the central chopping attachment into the main bowl of the food processor and add in the chunks of red cabbage. Pulse until chopped evenly. Tip into a waiting bowl.

2 Add in the broccoli and kale sprouts and repeat (they tend to be slightly more robust veg, so they may take a little longer to chop). Add to the mix.

3 Repeat with the beans and mangetout.

4 Place the vinegar, olive oil and a sprinkle of sea salt and sumac into a jam jar. Replace the lid and shake vigorously.

5 Pour the dressing over the slaw and mix well.

toppers

A piece of grilled salmon and a few blackberries makes this into an Instagram-worthy slaw.

morph your slaw
Stir-fried Purple Power with Bean Sprouts

1 Heat a little oil (I use coconut oil) in a pan or wok over a medium heat and add in a handful of washed, fresh bean sprouts. Stir to coat in the oil.

2 Add in any slaw and mix into the bean sprouts. Cook for 2–3 minutes, or until heated through.

3 Sprinkle over some dried chilli flakes and serve with a piece of cooked, flaked salmon.

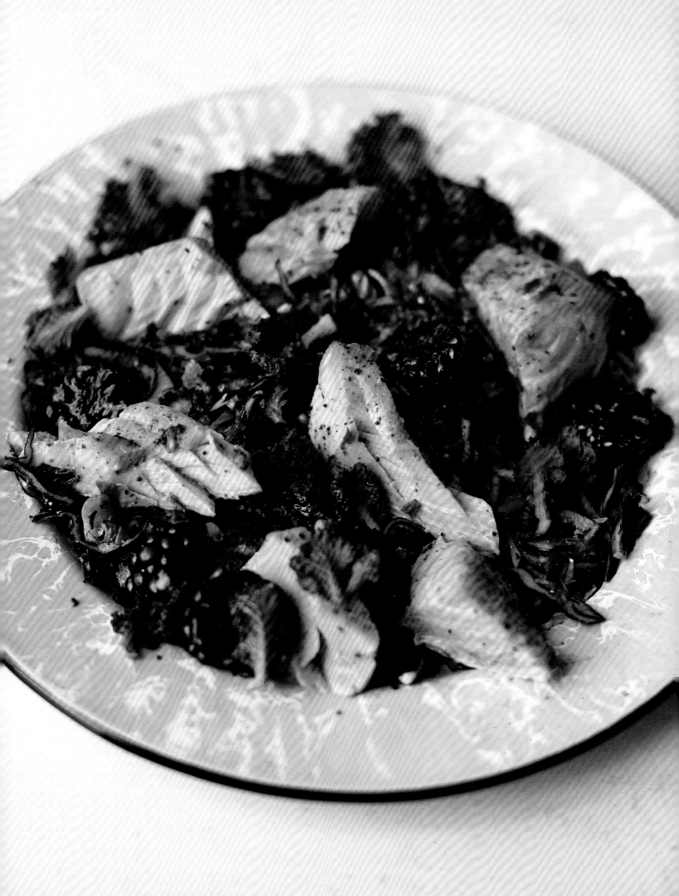

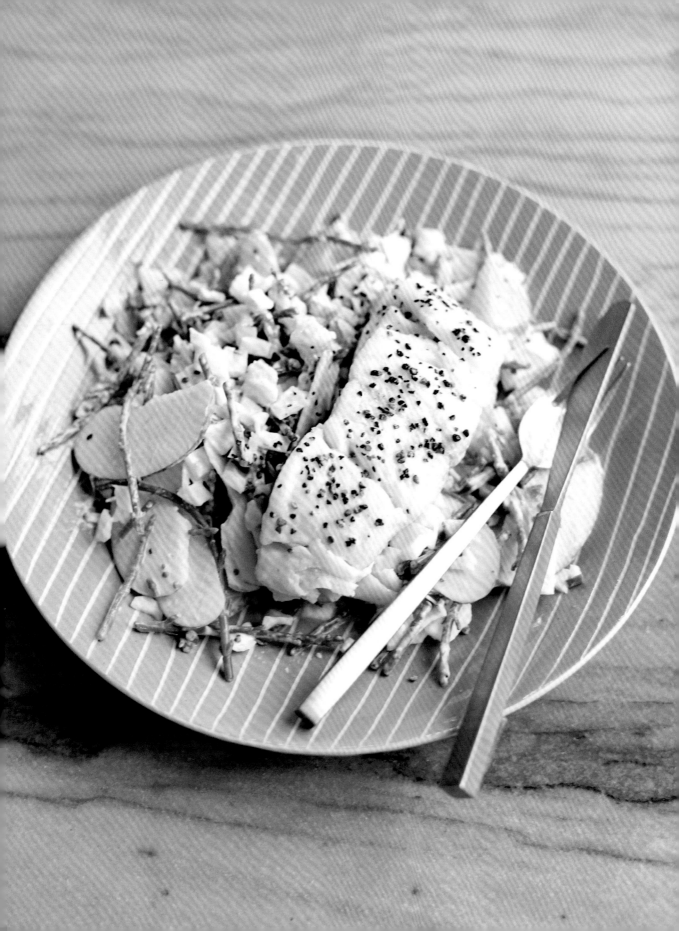

Applephire Slaw

Marsh samphire is a salty vegetable that grows on the sandy flats of tidal creeks and estuaries. It makes a valuable contribution to your mineral intake supplying magnesium, calcium, iron and zinc.

Most good fishmongers will stock samphire (best in season between June and August), although it has more recently become available in local supermarkets. Give the samphire a good soak and then rinse in water to reduce the saltiness.

150 g samphire
2 apples (I use Pink Lady, but any sweet apples will work well), cores removed
1 small sweet cabbage, core removed and chopped into quarters
Juice of 2 lemons
Sea salt

Makes 4 large portions

MORPH pictured

1 Place the central chopping attachment into the main bowl in the food processor and add in the samphire and apples. Pulse gently until chopped into small pieces. Add to a waiting bowl.

2 Next, add the cabbage. Repeat the pulse until finely shredded.

3 Mix the ingredients together and squeeze over the lemon juice and a sprinkle of sea salt. Mix together well.

toppers

This slaw has almost no fat in it. To help absorb the maximum nutritional potential, sprinkle with some omega-rich seeds. A sunflower and pumpkin seed mix brings a nice texture and crunch.

morph your slaw

Baked Fish with Potato Applephire Salad

1 Bake a piece of hake for 20 minutes at 180°C.

2 Meanwhile, boil a couple of handfuls of baby new potatoes until soft, about 12–15 minutes.

3 Drain the potatoes and chop into quarters.

4 Mix a couple of tablespoons of Greek yoghurt with a teaspoon of wholegrain mustard and add it to the slaw with the cooled potato chunks.

5 Top with the baked fish and season well.

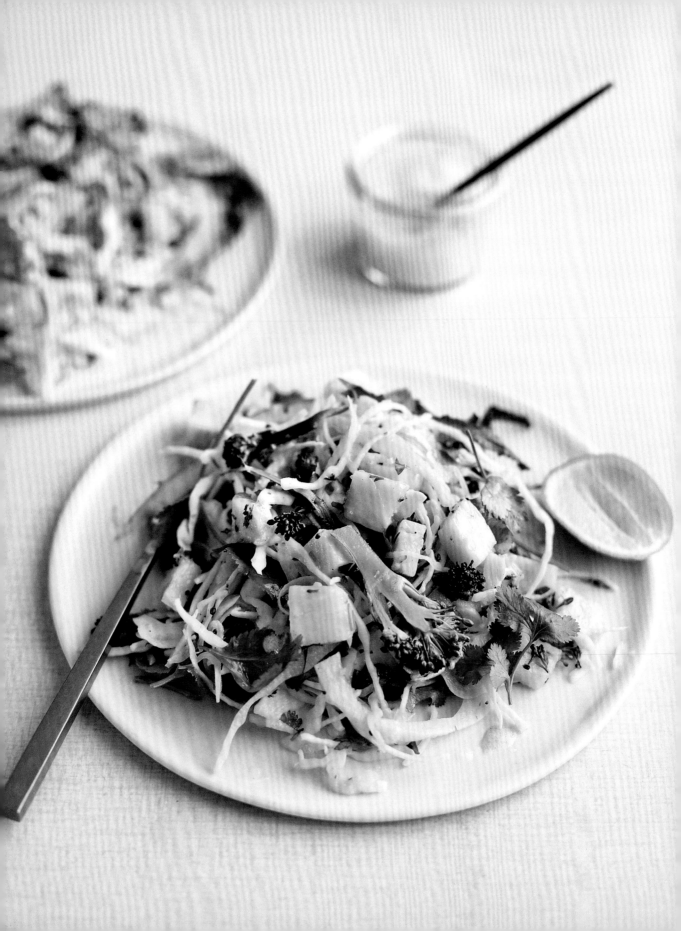

Pineapple + Purple Broccoli Slaw

Pineapple contains a powerful enzyme called bromelain, which helps relieve inflammation. After a particularly bad childhood bout of tonsillitis, my GP's advice to my mother was to load up on pineapples, and I've been a bit of a pineapple addict ever since!

My slight obsession with freezing foods does appear to excel with fruits like pineapple. So if you have a particularly large fruit, pop the pineapple leftovers into the freezer (sliced into chunks) to use at a later date.

100 g purple sprouting broccoli
½ white cabbage, core removed
4 handfuls of coriander
½ small pineapple, chopped into small chunks
½ teaspoon Dijon mustard
Drizzle of olive oil
2–3 tablespoons cider vinegar
Sea salt
1 lime, halved

Makes 4 large portions

1 Place the central chopping attachment into the main bowl of the food processor and add the broccoli. Pulse until finely chopped into an almost powdery consistency and tip into a waiting bowl.
2 Add the cabbage and coriander. Repeat to a more chunky chop. Mix into the broccoli.
3 Add the pineapple chunks and mix into the vegetables.
4 Pour the mustard, olive oil, vinegar and a sprinkle of sea salt into an empty jam jar. Place the lid on and shake vigorously. Pour over the slaw.
5 Squeeze the juice of the lime over the mixture and stir.

toppers
Sunflower seeds add omega-rich fats.

morph your slaw
Salmon, Pineapple + Purple Broccoli Pitta

1 Liquidize or mash any leftover slaw until the pineapple is mushy.
2 Marinate a piece of uncooked salmon in the mix.
3 Bake the salmon at 180°C for 20 minutes or until cooked.
4 Serve in a pitta bread.

Super-Smoothie-Tasha Slaw

The inspiration behind this goes to the incredible Natasha Grindley and her work with the Heal for Real social media page, set up after her terminal diagnosis for stomach cancer. When Natasha was given a month left to live by doctors, she fought on through the most gruelling chemotherapy. She made huge changes to her diet and nutrition plans, favouring foods that she credits helped her body endure the treatment, allowing her another 2 years of life.

6–8 stalks of celery, cut into
  quarters
1 courgette
3 heads of little gem lettuce, cut
  into thirds
4 spring onions
2 handfuls (½ tub) of raspberries
1 teaspoon ground cinnamon
2–3 tablespoons red wine vinegar
½–1 teaspoon horseradish sauce
Drizzle of olive oil

Makes 4 large portions

1 Place the central chopping attachment into the bowl of the processor.
2 Place the celery pieces into the bowl and replace the lid. Pulse until thickly chopped, then tip into a waiting bowl.
3 Add the courgette and lettuce pieces to the food processor bowl and repeat. Add to the celery and mix.
4 Hand-chop the spring onions into fine slices and mix in.
5 Next, place the raspberries with the remainder of the ingredients, apart from the olive oil, into the food processor. Pulse until you have a thick 'smoothie' mix and the raspberries have been mushed. Pour over the slaw and mix well. The mixture will turn a lovely light pink colour.
6 Use the olive oil to add a little extra coating to the mix.

toppers

Top with pecans or pine nuts.

morph your slaw

Roasted Plum + Goat's Cheese Smoothie Slaw

1 Place stoned plums, sliced into halves, on a baking tray and sprinkle with cinnamon. Bake at 180°C for 10 minutes or until just cooked.
2 On a separate baking tray, grill a full round slice of goat's cheese until softened.
3 Layer the plums on top of the slaw and finally top with the melted goat's cheese.

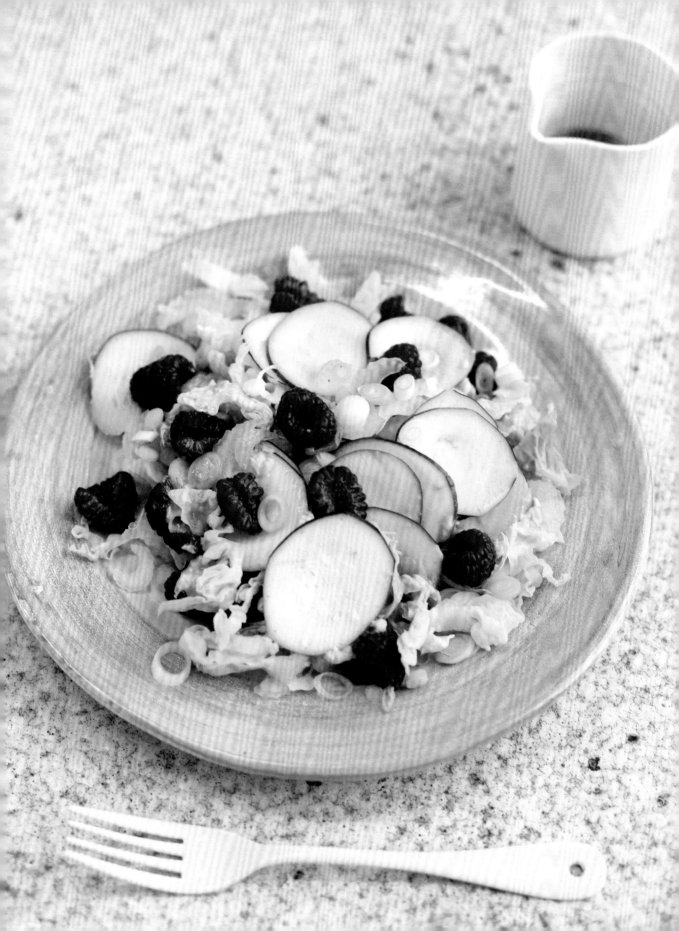

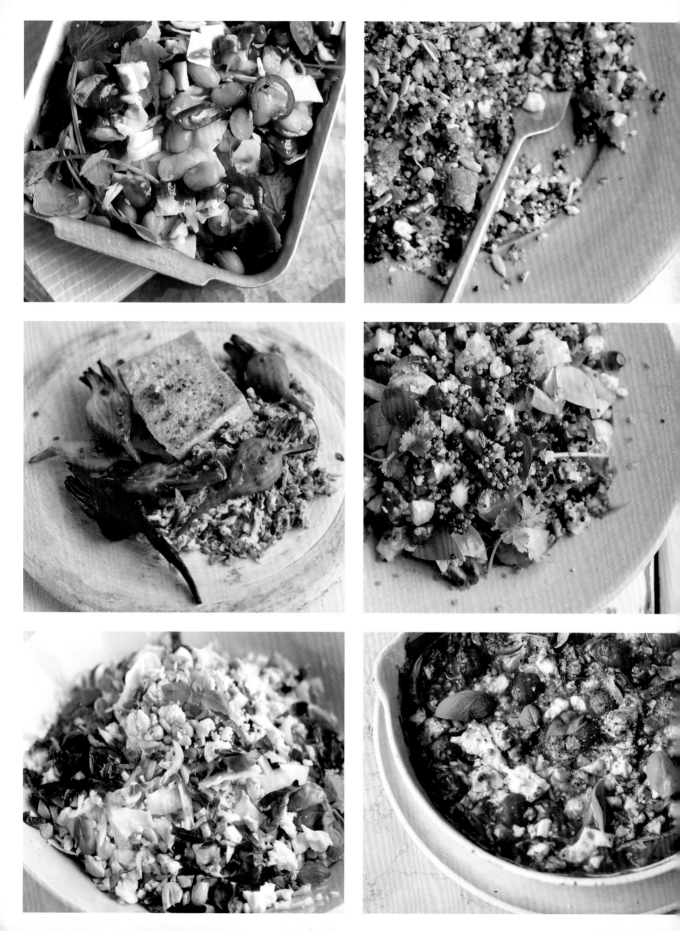

Energy Booster

Perfect for busy periods. One of the key deficits I see when working with diet-conscious clients is a lack of good-quality calories. In my experience, those looking to improve their health and fitness tend to cut macronutrients out of their diets too easily. Low-fat or low-carb diet fans lower their intake of good sources of fats and carbohydrates, overlooking that these are what fuel the body with the energy they need for fitness activities. Individual needs vary, and depend on how active you are each day. If you suffer from frequent energy slumps or fatigue, my top tip is to track what you are eating. Write it down! People are often surprised how little macronutrients they actually eat when they look back at their diet record. If after increasing your exercise levels you regularly suffer from sluggishness, try adding a little more macronutrient-dense food ingredients to your dishes.

Eating natural, nutrient-dense foods helps by providing a stable supply of energy. Research in this area is confusing and contradictory, so keep it simple. Keep natural sources of fat and carbohydrate in your eating plan. Try to aim for a balance, but be conscious that some days your energy needs will be greater than others. As a general rule of thumb, I tend to focus on higher levels of protein and fat on days when I am either moving less or moving at a slower rate. I keep higher carbohydrate meals for days when I am moving at higher intensities. Energy-lifting SuperSlaws and their serving suggestions work on this principle, so use them in accordance with your day-to-day needs, keeping your fuel stores at the ready for tasks ahead. Some of the higher calorie slaws were created on days when I knew I might be either missing a meal or not have time to break for fixed meals. For those struggling with regular hunger pangs, these Energy Booster SuperSlaws will help keep you satiated to stop you battling the temptations in that biscuit jar on the shelf!

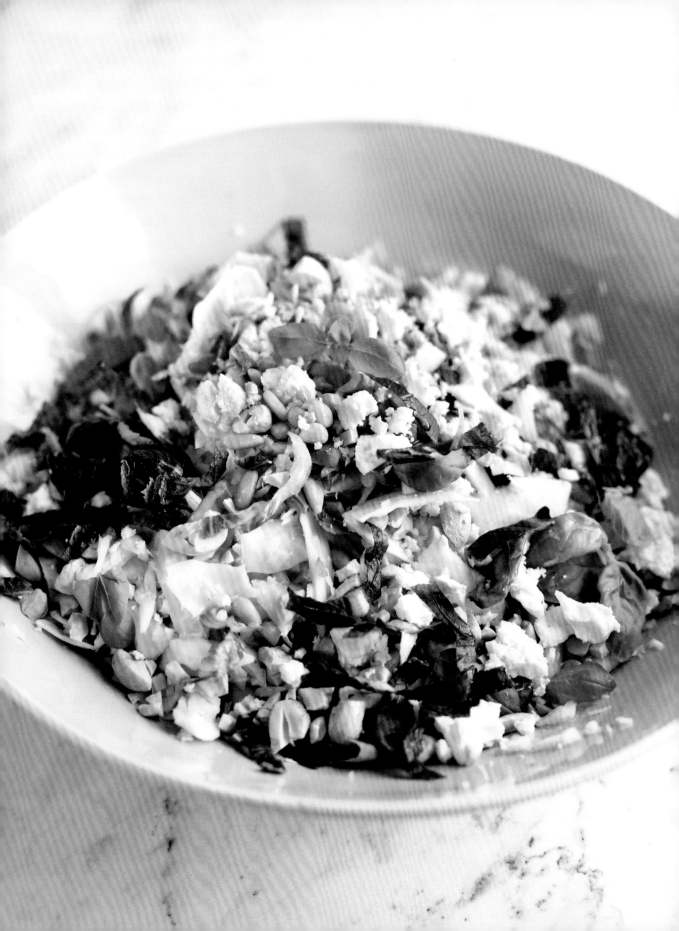

Pesto Punch Slaw

Pesto Punch is a cheese-lover's dream. Cheese gets a fairly bad reputation in most diet or nutrition plans, which often take a militant dairy approach. Most softer cheeses tend to be lower in fat and calories, but moderation as always is key. I have substituted the more traditional Parmesan flavour with feta, simply as this is slightly lower in calories (meaning you can put more in). Cottage cheese works well too, but does make the mixture fairly thick so you may have to add a little more oil.

1 small white cabbage, core removed and cut into large chunks
1 large handful of cashew nuts
1 large handful of basil leaves
1 head of chicory
1 small handful of pine nuts
⅓ block of feta cheese (you can use Parmesan for a more traditional pesto flavour)
Drizzle of olive oil

Makes 4 large portions

1 Place the central chopping attachment into the main bowl of the food processor and add the white cabbage.
2 Pulse until thickly chopped, then tip into a waiting bowl.
3 Add the cashew nuts and basil leaves and pulse until small pieces before adding to the cabbage in the bowl.
4 Repeat the above with the chicory head (this will take literally seconds to chop). Add to the mix and stir.
5 Sprinkle with the pine nuts and mix.
6 Now crumble in the feta (to keep your hands super-clean, break this up in the packet, then add in!).
7 Drizzle with the olive oil and mix.

toppers

For garlic-lovers, top with a little pan-fried or roasted garlic mixed into a few handfuls of cooked quinoa.

morph your slaw

Sweet Potato Pesto Burgers

1 Bake two large slices of sweet potato in a 200°C oven for 15 minutes.
2 Grill a good-quality beef, lamb or chicken burger for 3 minutes on each side, or until cooked.
3 Coat/layer the burger with leftover slaw.
4 Serve in between the sweet potato slices.

Nuts about Slaw

It goes without saying that I am nuts about slaw! I once received a message on social media that I may eat 'too much slaw', which I took as a compliment. I couldn't have got a more apt accolade that I practise what I preach! This is an energy-and-calorie dense dish, so you won't need much of it to feel full, and it will make a perfect snack for a busy day. You will notice this slaw contains no vegetables, but you can of course pair with a vegetable of your choice, or mix with another greens-based slaw.

1 large handful of walnuts
1 large handful of pecans
1 large handful of almonds
1 large handful of cashew nuts
1 large handful of dried coconut
1 small handful of prunes
1 small handful of dried apricots
150 g pre-cooked quinoa (this can be bought in packets from most supermarkets)
Juice of 1 orange
Sunflower seeds
Sea salt

Makes 4 large portions

1 Place the central chopping attachment into the main bowl of the food processor.
2 Place all of the ingredients (except the quinoa, orange juice and seeds) into the main bowl. Be warned this will be a noisy blitz, so hold the lid on tightly! Pulse/chop into roughly even pieces and place in a waiting bowl.
3 Add the cooked quinoa.
4 Squeeze over the juice of the orange.
5 Sprinkle with the sunflower seeds and a sprinkle of sea salt and mix.

toppers

For a savoury protein boost, add cottage cheese

morph your slaw
Chocolate Protein Nut Smoothie Bowl

1 Mix any leftover slaw with a scoop of chocolate-flavoured protein powder.
2 Add a few scoops of Greek yoghurt, a little almond milk and a banana.
3 Blitz together in the food processor.
4 Serve in a bowl with a few mixed berries, a shaving of dark chocolate or a drizzle of honey.

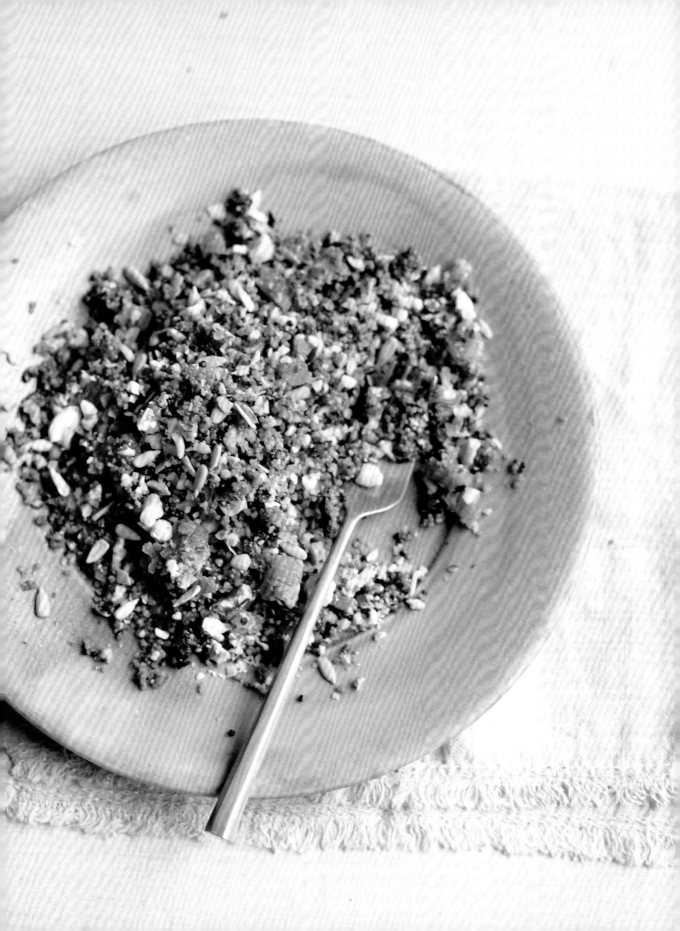

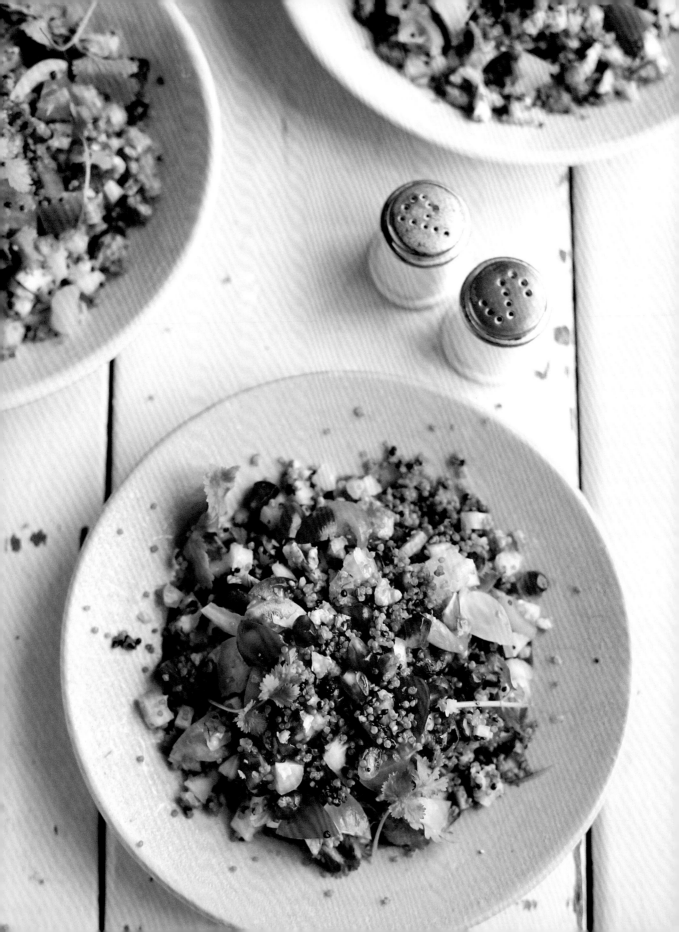

Quinoa Crackle Slaw

There are mixed reports about the good and the bad of grains. I once gave grains up for a long period and I have to say having reintroduced them into my diet I have much more energy. The quality of the grain is important, however. Quinoa is probably the most popular "grain" in the health-enthusiast's armour, as it holds an unusually high ratio of protein to carbohydrates (compared with other grains). This is because it is technically a seed and not a true grain. Full of fibre, it adds bulk to any meal. If you aren't a fan, use pre-cooked couscous, bulgur wheat or rice.

10 stalks of celery, thinly sliced
1 large handful of coriander, roughly chopped
1 handful of walnuts
150 g pre-cooked quinoa or alternative grains
1 lemon, halved
Drizzle of olive oil
Sea salt
1 pomegranate, deseeded or 2 packets (100 g) of pomegranate seeds (see page 30)

Makes 4 large portions

1 Mix together the celery and coriander.
2 Crush the walnuts using either a pestle and mortar or by placing into a robust food bag and bashing with a rolling pin.
3 Mix all of the ingredients together and add the pre-cooked grains.
4 Squeeze the juice of the lemon halves over the mix.
5 Add the olive oil and coat the mixture.
6 Sprinkle with sea salt and the pomegranate seeds to garnish.

toppers

Hand-chopped tomatoes make a delicious TOPPER, providing the dish with a tabbouleh salad vibe.

morph your slaw
Quinoa Crackle Pizza

1 Take any leftover slaw and place in the food processor with a little extra cooked quinoa, a pinch of salt and a pinch of baking powder. Blend consistently until it becomes a thick, creamy paste. You may need to add a little water if it becomes too heavy.
2 Line a baking tin with baking paper and pour in the mixture. Bake in a 200°C oven for 15–20 minutes until golden, then turn for an extra 5–10 minutes.
3 Top your pizza base with your choice of tomatoes/veggies/meats or cheese and bake further as required.

Spicy Texas Slaw

This is a spicy slaw topped fantastically with mixed beans. Beans provide a great protein source and are also fibre and carbohydrate-rich – perfect for adding a little extra 'bulk'. For those who don't tolerate beans well, adding a little pre-cooked rice into this slaw at the end will help provide a carbohydrate-rich alternative. This is another easy slaw to whip up without a food processor.

2 large handfuls of coriander, roughly chopped
3 handfuls of watercress, roughly chopped
1 small white cabbage, core removed
2 tablespoons natural yoghurt or quark
2–3 red chillies, deseeded and thinly sliced
2–3 tablespoons olive oil
1 tablespoon ground cumin
1 teaspoon hot chilli sauce
Sea salt

Makes 4 large portions

TOPPER pictured

1 Mix the coriander and watercress together.

2 Finely chop the white cabbage and add.

3 Spoon in the yoghurt or quark and then add the chilli and mix well.

4 Add the olive oil, cumin, chilli sauce and sea salt to a jam jar. Place the lid on and shake vigorously. Add to the slaw and mix well.

toppers

A few handfuls of broad beans, podded and boiled for a few minutes or a small tin of kidney beans.

morph your slaw

Texas Chilli

1 Pan-fry some lean mince until brown, about 5–6 minutes.

2 Add in the slaw and pan-fry for 3–4 minutes.

3 Serve with cooked basmati rice or quinoa.

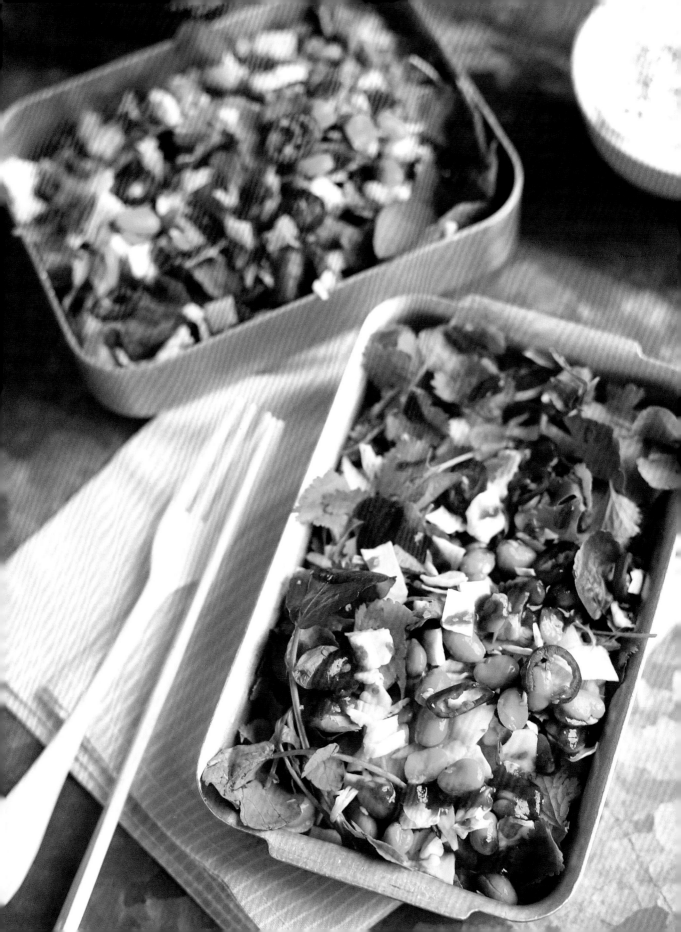

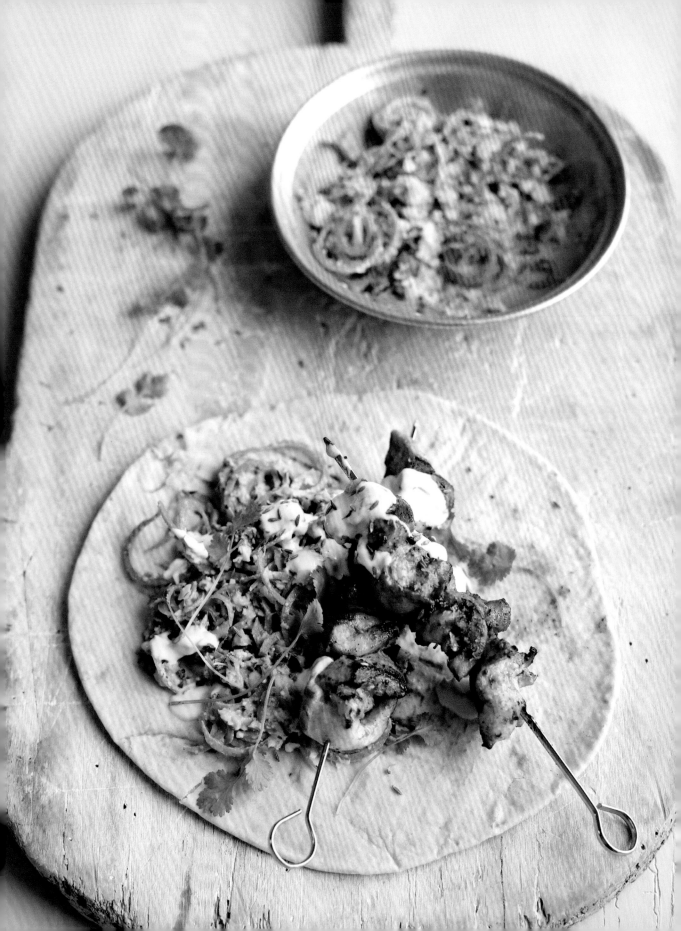

Hummus Slaw

Hummus is a staple in most fridges these days and a way of adding some protein and good fats to dishes. For an extra Middle Eastern feel, add purple olives or dry-cured black olives.

In the Middle Ages, cumin seed was thought to enhance love and fidelity, so it is said to have been carried by wedding guests as a sign of luck. It has a pungent flavour, which works well with tahini and chickpeas.

1 broccoli, cut into quarters
2 courgettes
6 olives (black or purple)
3 carrots
1 tablespoon wholegrain mustard
2 tablespoons olive oil
2 tablespoons hummus
4 tablespoons cider vinegar
½ teaspoon ground cumin
Sea salt

Makes 4 large portions

MORPH pictured

1 Place the central chopping attachment into the bowl of the processor.
2 Place the broccoli in the bowl and replace the lid. Pulse until thickly chopped, then tip into a waiting bowl.
3 Add the courgettes and olives and pulse until small chunky pieces before adding to the broccoli in the bowl.
4 Next, change your chopping tool to the flat 'chopper' blade. If you prefer, you can chop by hand, grater or a spiralizer for a lovely ribbon effect. Feed the carrots into the opening at the top while turning the food processor on until thinly sliced. Add to the mix.
5 Put the mustard, olive oil, hummus and vinegar into an empty jam jar. Place the lid on and shake vigorously. This will be a thick consistency – if you need to thin it, add a little more vinegar.
6 Pour over the slaw and mix well. Sprinkle with the cumin and sea salt.

toppers

Balance this higher fat dish by TOPPING with a lean protein source, such as fish, turkey or chicken.

morph your slaw
Hummus Kebab

1 Pan-fry cubed chicken pieces for 5–7 minutes, or skewer the meat and grill for 8 minutes.
2 Pile the slaw and chicken on to a flat bread.
3 Top with natural yoghurt and a sprinkle of cumin.

Cauliflower Feta Slaw

This slaw is the perfect solution for any cauliflower cheese lovers out there. Cauliflower is a versatile vegetable that is often bland or overcooked, so I wanted to try and give it a little more appeal. I think feta works well, but swap for your cheese of choice.

A great way to help with portion control is to mix this with a small amount of plain rice.

1 medium cauliflower, core removed and cut into small florets
1 medium iceberg lettuce, finely shredded (you can do this by hand or in the food processor)
1 green chilli, deseeded
3 cm cube of fresh ginger, peeled (minced ginger can also be used)
¼ block of feta cheese
2–3 tablespoons cider vinegar
3–4 tablespoons olive oil
Himalayan pink sea salt

Makes 4 large portions

1 Place the central chopping attachment in the main bowl of the food processor and add the cauliflower florets. Pulse gently until they form small, chunky pieces (if you want to make this into a rice-type consistency, just pulse a little longer). Dependent on the size of your cauliflower you may need to do this in stages. Add to a waiting bowl.

2 Mix in the finely shredded iceberg.

3 Finely hand-chop the chilli and ginger and add in.

4 Crumble the feta cheese over the mix.

5 Add the vinegar, olive oil and sea salt to a jam jar. Place the lid on and shake vigorously. Pour over the slaw and mix well.

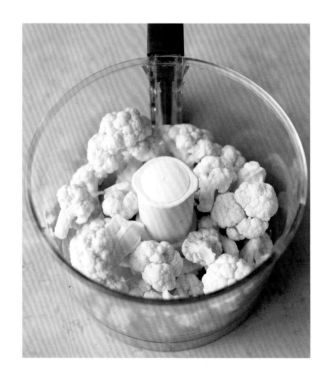

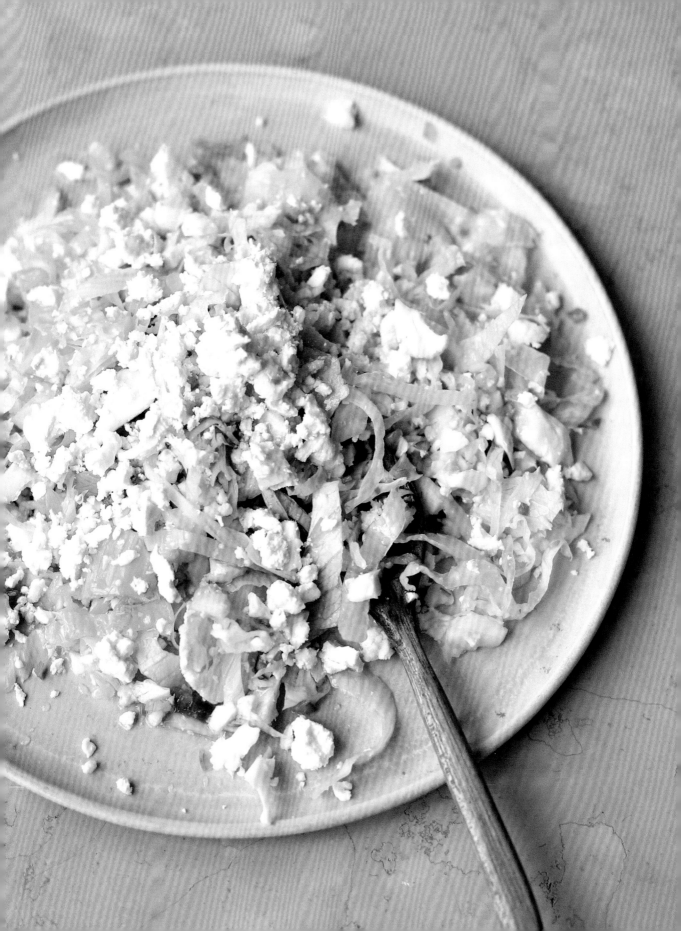

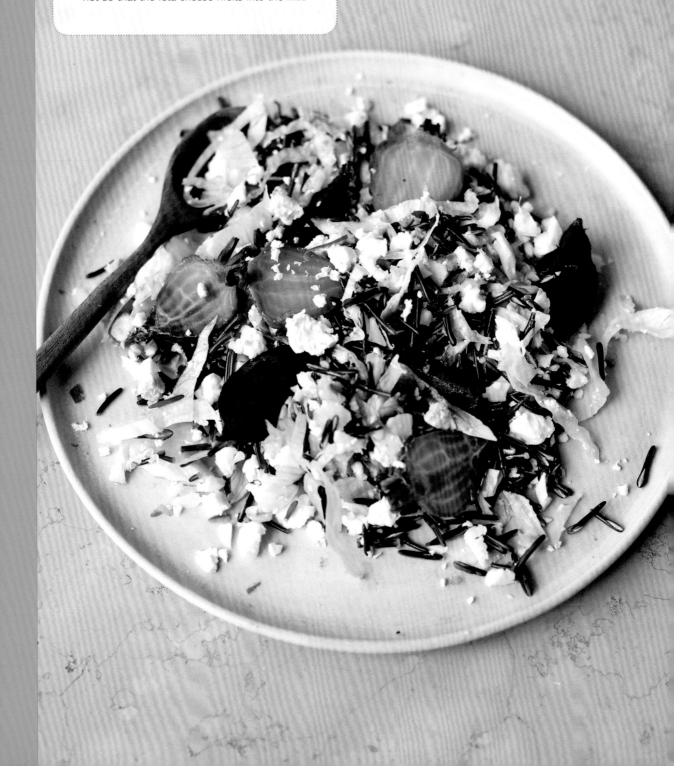

toppers

Adding a carbohydrate, such as some cooked rice or roasted beetroot, helps to add a little starch to this fibre-rich slaw. Mix while the rice or beetroot is still hot so that the feta cheese melts into the mix.

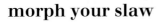

morph your slaw

Creamy Cauliflower, Feta + Tomato Bake

1 Place a 400g tin of chopped cherry tomatoes in a bowl and mix together with any leftover slaw. Transfer to a baking dish.

2 Preheat the oven to 180°C and place in the middle of the oven for 15–20 minutes.

3 Drizzle over a tablespoon of creamy full-fat Greek yoghurt, some basil leaves and serve.

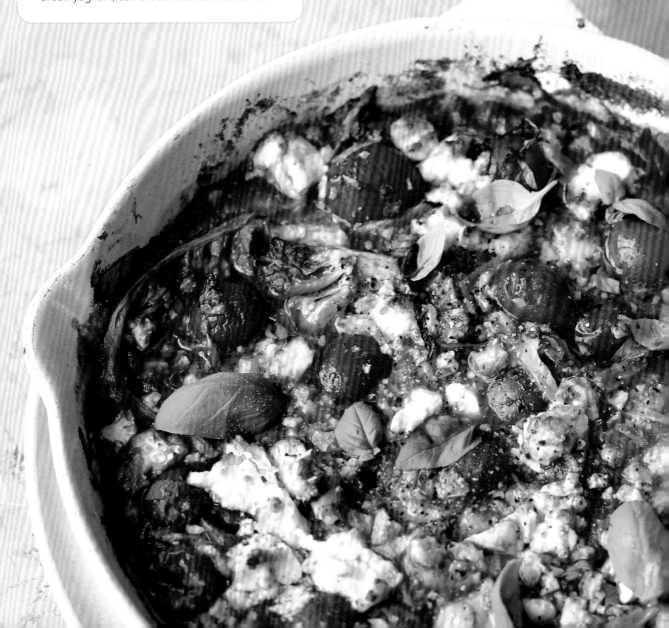

Broc-a-Mole Slaw

I've introduced my SuperSlaw twists to an avocado classic as I am yet to meet anyone who does not like guacamole. I am also yet to meet anyone who can't eat a very large serving in one (without thinking about excess calories or other nutrients being squeezed into their meal). Fat is highly satiating, so adding veggies into a high-fat dish is an easy way to make sure you balance some additional fibre with calorie-dense meals. This can be prepared as a more conventional salad, with a dressing on the side or it can all be blitzed to create a more traditional guacamole. Both are delicious, so make whichever version you wish!

1 large head (400 g) of broccoli,
   chopped into pieces
1 bag (150 g) of sugar snap peas
1 extra large or 2 smaller avocados
6–8 pitted green olives
3 tablespoons sun-dried tomatoes
1 red chilli, deseeded
1 lemon, halved
Sea salt
Dash of olive oil

Makes 4 large portions

1 For a guacamole style slaw, place the central chopping attachment in the main bowl of the food processor, followed by the broccoli pieces. Replace the lid and pulse gently until chopped into consistently sized small chunks. Remove any bigger pieces and repeat. For a more textured slaw, use a mandolin to thinly slice the broccoli pieces. Add the mixture to a waiting bowl.

2 Repeat the processing with the sugar snap peas, pulsing for just seconds to avoid over-chopping, or hand-slice into strips.

3 Add the avocado, olives and sun-dried tomatoes to the food processor. Whizz until the mixture is thick and smooth. Mix into the blitzed veggies or place in a small bowl on the side.

4 Slice the red chilli and add to the vegetable mix.

5 Squeeze the lemon juice over the vegetables and add a sprinkle of sea salt. Taste the dressing and then add olive oil to drizzle and to thin out the mixture if needed.

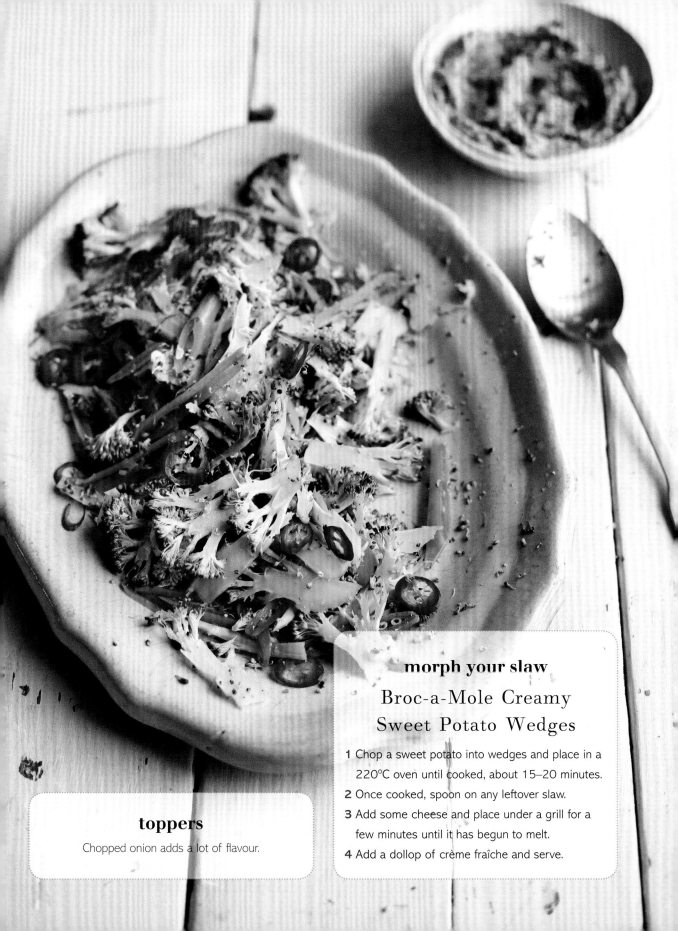

morph your slaw
Broc-a-Mole Creamy Sweet Potato Wedges

1 Chop a sweet potato into wedges and place in a 220°C oven until cooked, about 15–20 minutes.

2 Once cooked, spoon on any leftover slaw.

3 Add some cheese and place under a grill for a few minutes until it has begun to melt.

4 Add a dollop of crème fraîche and serve.

toppers
Chopped onion adds a lot of flavour.

Peanut Satay Slaw

Nut butters are now widely available, acknowledged as a healthy source of fuel (fat) and protein. Look out for brands that sell the butter in its purist form (preferably 100 percent pure). That way you avoid controversial ingredients such as palm oil or a high salt (sodium) content. The nut butter and peanuts makes it higher in fat and satiating, while the chestnuts provide an energy boost, perfect for anyone who has a long day ahead.

1 large bag (250 g) of bean sprouts, steamed for 2–4 minutes
1 bag (150g) of green beans
1 bag (150 g) of mangetout
1–2 red chillies, deseeded
1 small cube of fresh ginger, peeled
1 small handful of Thai basil
3–4 handfuls of drained water chestnuts
2–3 tablespoons balsamic vinegar
1 tablespoon peanut butter or any other nut butter
Sea salt
3–4 tablespoons peanuts

Makes 4 large portions

1 Run the bean sprouts under cold water after you have steamed them. Roughly hand-chop and layer on to a large flat plate.
2 Place the remainder of the vegetables and herbs, apart from the water chestnuts, into the main bowl of the food processor with the central chopping attachment. Pulse gently until they form small, chunky pieces.
3 Mix the veg into the chopped bean sprouts.
4 Chop the water chestnuts in half by hand and add to the mix.
5 Add the vinegar, peanut butter and a sprinkle of sea salt to a jam jar. Place the lid on and shake vigorously. Nut butters vary a lot in consistency. If the mixture is too thick, you can stir with a teaspoon or add in a little more vinegar.
6 Add the dressing to the slaw and mix well.
7 Season with the peanuts.

toppers

Dehydrated or oven-baked kale makes a nice extra-green crunch to this nutty fusion.

morph your slaw
Peanut Satay Noodles

1 Cook a handful of rice vermicelli noodles according to the packet instructions.
2 Mix the noodles with any leftover slaw.
3 Top with a piece of cooked chicken or fish for a full macronutrient plate.

Avocado Kale Slaw

Another SuperSlaw avocado twist classic! Avocado Kale Slaw has a slightly lower fat content than the Broc-a-Mole sister slaw. This is a fantastic way to convert any kale haters by secretly creeping in this nutrient-rich leafy green into a hidden base of avocado loveliness. Great for trying to convince children to eat a few extra veggies without having to cover everything in sauce! The MORPH allows you to add even more vegetables into a hidden wrap – perfect for lunch boxes or snacks. I won't tell if you don't…

250 g kale
¼ red onion
1 garlic clove
1 green chilli, deseeded
4 small or 2 medium avocados
1 lemon, halved
½ teaspoon smoked paprika
Sea salt
Drizzle of olive oil

Makes 4 large portions

1 Place the central chopping attachment into the main bowl of the food processor, followed by the kale. Replace the lid and blitz until the kale is finely chopped. You may need to do this in batches. Place in a waiting bowl.

2 Repeat the above with the red onion, garlic, chilli and avocados until the mixture is thick. Alternatively, to ensure an 'even slice', you may want to chop the garlic and chilli by hand.

3 Squeeze with lemon juice and sprinkle with paprika and salt. Taste and add olive oil to drizzle and thin out the mixture a little if needed.

toppers

Chopped sun-dried tomatoes.

morph your slaw

Avocado Kale Spinach Wrap

1 Layer a wrap with spinach, tomatoes and any leftover slaw.

2 Top with a sliced cooked chicken fillet.

3 Roll into wraps and serve.

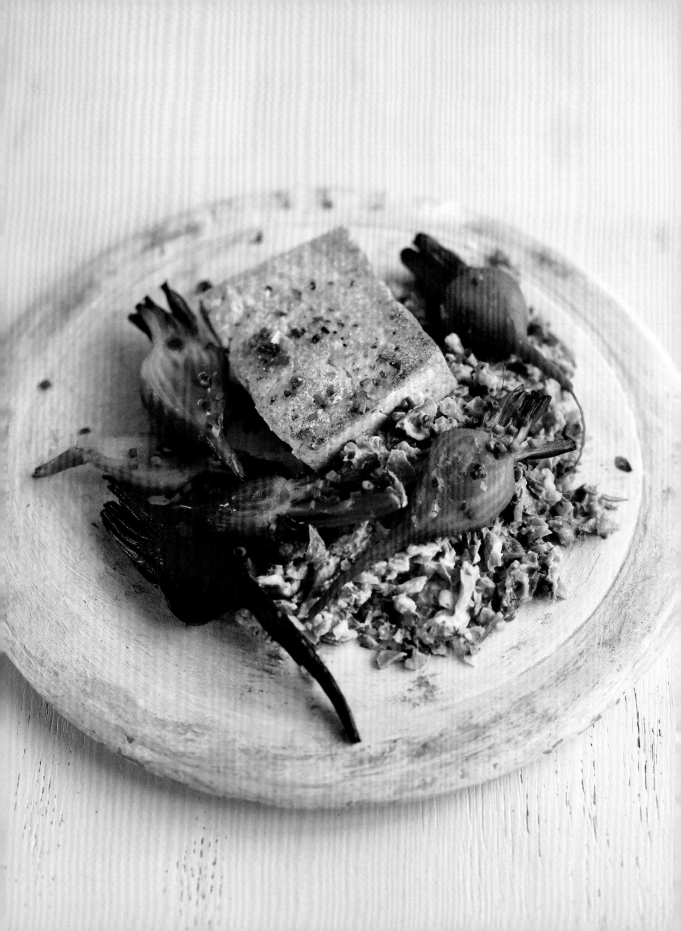

Green Garden Slaw

Created after a wonderful donation of greens from my dad's home-grown vegetable patch. Garden Slaw helped utilize a mass production of mangetout! A good source of vitamins C, K, B1 and potassium, mangetout hold an abundance of nutrients while remaining low in calories. This allows a higher fat dressing to be perfectly paired with this slaw. If you are tracking calories closely or are pairing this slaw with a particularly higher fat protein source, you can always use lower-fat sources of yoghurt and hummus within the recipe.

1½ bags (250 g) of mangetout
1 handful of chives
4 handfuls of parsley
8 pitted olives (I used green Greek olives)
1 lime, halved
2 heaped tablespoons full-fat Greek yoghurt
2 heaped tablespoons full-fat hummus
Dash of olive oil
Sea salt

Makes 4 large portions

MORPH pictured

1 Place the central chopping attachment into the main bowl of the food processor, followed by the mangetout and the chives. Replace the lid and pulse gently until chopped.

2 Add the parsley and olives and repeat until they are slightly 'mushy'. Tip into a waiting jam jar.

3 Juice the lime directly into the jar and add the yoghurt, hummus, a dash of olive oil and a sprinkle of salt. Shake vigorously with the lid on until mixed. The mixture will be thick – add a little more olive oil if you need to for consistency.

4 Pour over the vegetables and mix well.

toppers

Top with flax or cumin seeds for a super crunch.

morph your slaw

Roasted Vegetable Garden Slaw with Tofu

1 Cut the tofu, carrot and beetroot into cubes.

2 Bake at 200°C until cooked, about 15 minutes.

3 Transfer to a bowl and mix in the slaw.

4 Serve with a side of pre-cooked bulgur wheat.

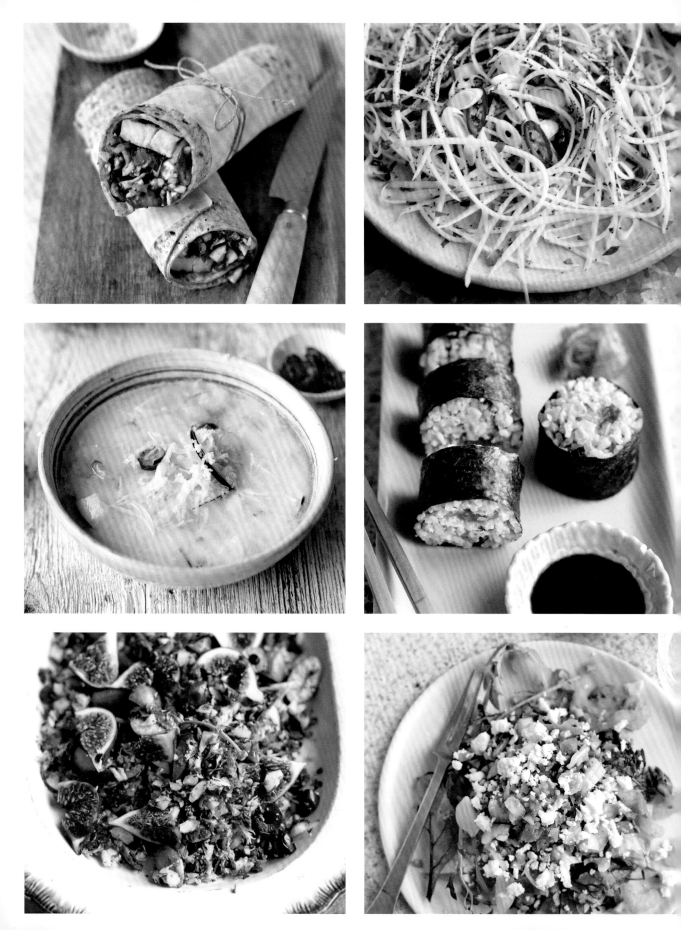

Revitalize

It's fairly common knowledge that too much sugar, alcohol and caffeine can not only cause depressive symptoms and fluctuating moods, but also lead to a dull complexion or hormonal breakouts. Science suggests this all links with the release of toxins and cortisol (the stress hormone) within the body. The skin is an organ that requires constant regeneration, so we should feed it in the best way we can to aid in this process.

I wanted to produce a mix of ingredients that help you feel like you have a glowing complexion from the inside, without trying to bamboozle anyone with pseudo-scientific ingredients. Revitalizing nutrients will help your skin shine by mixing large amounts of key skin health vitamins (A, B, C and E) with plenty of healthy fats, which are also known to be hugely beneficial for the plump and hydrated appearance of skin. Serving recommendations and toppers are all based around this principle, but don't forget to top up with a good helping of beauty sleep! As with mind and body, skin repair happens most efficiently when you sleep.

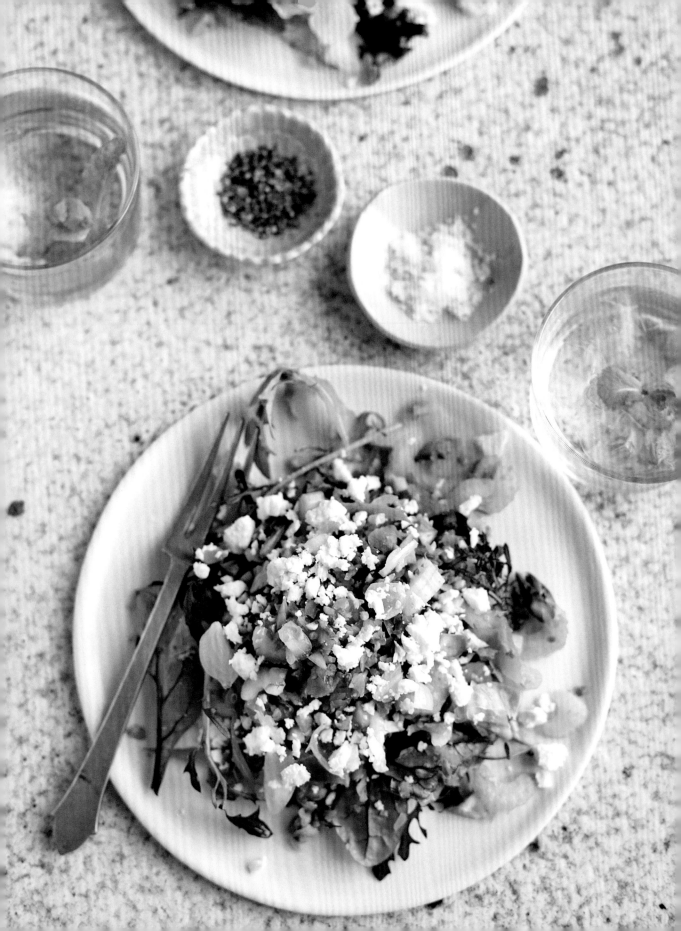

Fresh + Pickle Slaw

Who would have thought cheese and pickle could be good for you?
Celery is full of anti-inflammatory health benefits, including its protection
against inflammation in the digestive tract. It helps keep your immune
system boosted with vitamin C, and has a high water content so aids
rehydration. It also holds silica, a magical element linked with skin, hair
and nail health.

1 bunch (150 g) of asparagus,
woody ends removed
6–8 stalks of celery
1 bag (150 g) of sugar snap peas
8–10 pickled silverskin onions,
drained (if you only have the
larger ones, just use less)
½ bag (75–100 g) of pre-mixed
leaves (any you can find!)
¼–½ block of feta cheese (if eating
as a main meal, I add in more
cheese)
1 lime, halved
2–4 tablespoons olive oil
Sea salt

Makes 4 large portions

1 Blanch the asparagus by cooking for 2 minutes in boiling water, then cool by running under cold water.
2 Add the flat 'chopper' blade to the top of the food processor. Replace the lid. Place the celery into the opening at the top while turning the food processor on. Push it through with the added attachment until finely sliced (you can do this by hand if you prefer).
3 Next, change the blades over so the central chopping attachment is in place. Add the sugar snap peas with the pickled onions. Pulse gently until small, chunky pieces form.
4 Mix in with the celery.
5 Repeat the chop with the asparagus and leaves and mix into the celery.
6 Crumble the cheese over the top and squeeze over the juice of the lime.
7 Drizzle over olive oil to taste.
8 Season with sea salt and mix well.

toppers

Mini new potatoes turn this slaw into a quirky alternative to a potato salad and is perfect for bbqs!

morph your slaw

Easy Cheesy Pickle Fish Slaw Cakes

1 Mix any leftover Pickle Slaw with cooked fish (such as tinned tuna or salmon) and add a raw egg to help bind it together.
2 Roll into balls, then flatten into cake shapes. Coat in a little flour if too sticky.
3 Pan-fry or grill for 4 minutes on each side.

Fruity Fennel Slaw

I am not a natural fennel lover. I find it has quite an overpowering taste, however, in the interest of trying to diversify my vegetable taste buds, I began to experiment. Adding a little fruit transforms this vegetable to produce a beautifully relaxed flavour, which has turned this into one of my favourite slaws. A fabulous slaw MORPH for this dish adds in a little nut butter to turn it into a whole new flavour. Fennel is a great source of collagen-building vitamin C and heart-friendly potassium.

1 small head of fennel, ends cut off
    and sliced lengthways
200 g kale
2 'just ripe' pears
2–3 tablespoons olive oil
1 tablespoon white balsamic vinegar
Juice of 1 lemon
Sea salt

Makes 4 large portions

1 Add the flat 'chopper' blade to the top of the food processor. Replace the lid. Place the fennel slices into the opening at the top while turning the food processor on. Push them through with the added attachment until finely sliced. Once chopped, place into a waiting bowl.

2 Next, change the blades over so the central chopping attachment is in place. Add the kale and pulse chop in batches. Add to the fennel.

3 Add the pears and chop until they form fine pieces. Stir into the rest of the mix.

4 Add the olive oil, vinegar, lemon juice and a sprinkle of sea salt to a jam jar. Place the lid on and shake vigorously.

5 Pour over the slaw and mix well.

toppers

Add a handful of chopped walnuts.

morph your slaw
Nut Butter
Fruity Fennel

1 Stir a spoonful of nut butter into the slaw.
2 Mix well and serve.

Tahini + Lemon Slaw

Made from raw sesame seeds and found in many Asian dishes, tahini is an excellent source of skin-friendly fatty acids. It has an unusual flavour, which is fabulous with green veg and a hint of lemon. It's another great way to spice up plain veggies in a super-quick fashion. Tahini is a thick mixture, so make sure you shake the slaw and mix it well to combine the ingredients.

1 large Chinese leaf cabbage, sliced
200 g kale
2–3 tablespoons white wine vinegar
1 lemon, halved
3 tablespoons tahini
Sea salt

Makes 4 large portions

1 Place the central chopping attachment into the main bowl of the food processor.
2 Place the Chinese leaf into the main bowl and pulse until chunkily chopped. This will take literally seconds. Pour into a waiting bowl.
3 Repeat this with the kale. You may need to do this in stages. Add to the Chinese leaf.
4 Add the vinegar, lemon, tahini and a sprinkle of sea salt to a jam jar. Place the lid on and shake vigorously. Tahini is quite a thick consistency, so you may need a little more shake than normal. Add in a little extra vinegar if you find it too thick. Pour over the slaw and mix well.

toppers

Add a sprinkle of cumin and some chopped cucumber.

morph your slaw

Tahini + Lemon Slaw Mash with Mackerel

1 Pop any leftover slaw into a food processor and blend until a smoother consistency.
2 Mix in with pre-cooked mashed potato.
3 Serve with mackerel fillets.

SuperHero Slaw

SuperHero Slaw was born after I hit the kitchen feeling tired, but creative. I had been given a huge amount of raw cacao, which, to be honest, I wasn't sure what to do with! I'm not a natural baker, but having heard so much about the antioxidant benefits I wanted to introduce it into a slaw to see if it would work in a vegetable dish – and I wasn't disappointed with a winning sweet-and-sour flavour. Apparently it has up to four times the antioxidants of green tea, but without the bitter aftertaste.

200 g spinach
150 g broccoli, cut into quarters
10–12 radishes, topped and tailed
10 pitted purple olives (I use Kalamata)
10 caper berries, stems removed
2–3 tablespoons balsamic vinegar
1 tablespoon raw cacao powder
½ teaspoon sweet chilli sauce
1–2 tablespoons olive oil
Sea salt

Makes 4 large portions

TOPPER pictured

1 Place the central chopping attachment into the main bowl of the food processor.
2 Place the spinach and broccoli into the main bowl. Pulse gently until small, chunky pieces form. You may need to do this in stages.
3 Next, add the radishes and olives and pulse until chopped and resembling a chunky paste.
4 Chop the caper berries by hand into halves and add to the mix.
5 Add the vinegar, cacao powder, sweet chilli sauce, olive oil and sea salt to a jam jar. Place the lid on and shake vigorously. If the mixture is too thick you can stir with a teaspoon or add in a little more vinegar.
6 Add to the slaw and mix well.

toppers

Quartered figs will give this slaw a lovely sweetness.

morph your slaw
Superhero Fruit Salad

1 Chop a kiwi, apple and a pear into cubes.
2 Mix in a few handfuls of leftover slaw.
3 Sprinkle with nuts, seeds and a dollop of crème fraîche.

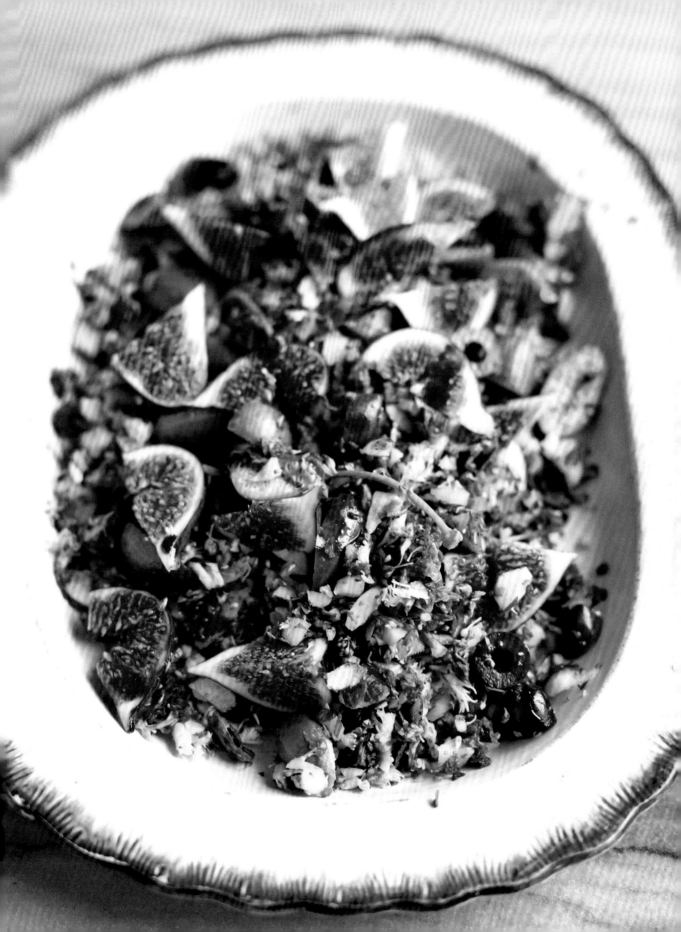

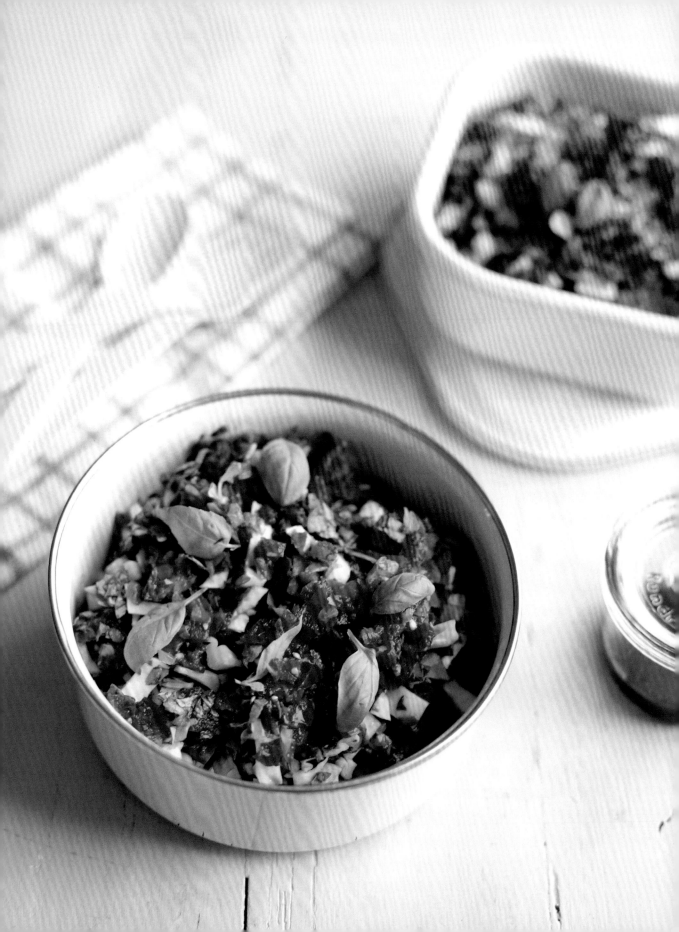

Salsa Slaw

Orange and red vegetables are full of beta-carotene, which (converted to vitamin A) helps prevent against premature ageing and cell damage. If you can't track down an orange variety of tomato, miniature red ones will be just as good. Spinach is also naturally high in betacarotene (vitamin A), so throwing in a little extra spinach greens into this slaw will help give you an extra radiance boost!

1 sweet red pepper, deseeded and any core removed
1 full tub (75 g) of mini orange tomatoes
1 large handful of Greek basil leaves
1 large handful of spinach
1 large handful of mixed green cabbage leaves (I use pre-shredded ones in packets from the local supermarket)
3–4 tablespoons balsamic vinegar
2–3 tablespoons olive oil
Sea salt

Makes 4 large portions

1 Place the central chopping attachment into the main bowl of the food processor.

2 Place the red pepper and tomatoes into the main bowl and pulse very lightly until chopped. This will take literally seconds. Try to avoid pulsing too hard as the ingredients will go mushy due to their high water content. Pour into a waiting bowl.

3 Repeat this with the basil, spinach and cabbage leaves until finely chopped. Mix in with the tomatoes and pepper.

4 Add the vinegar, olive oil and sea salt to a jam jar. Place the lid on and shake vigorously. Pour over the slaw and mix well.

morph your slaw

Stuffed Peppers with Anchovies + Salsa Slaw

1 Slice 2 peppers into halves and hollow out any core and seeds.

2 Stuff the peppers with leftover slaw and a few slices of chopped garlic.

3 Place mini anchovy fillets over the top.

4 Drizzle with a dash of balsamic vinegar.

5 Bake in a 180°C oven until the peppers are cooked, about 25 minutes.

6 Garnish with basil leaves and serve.

toppers

Toasted pine nuts.

Provence Slaw

Olives are easily available and contain an unusually good mix of both antioxidants and healthy fats. With a bitter, but zesty taste, they pair really well with the concentrated flavour of sun-dried tomatoes. If you want to save a little on the olives and tomatoes, look out for olive and tomato mixes, sold in jars, but check the dressing they come in (look out for an olive oil marinade). If you find an olive-tomato mix marinated in a herby dressing, you can add a small amount of this to your slaw as well. For a little variation, try steaming the cauliflower for a few minutes first.

1 medium cauliflower
8–10 stalks of celery
1 bag (150–200 g) of mangetout
12 large mixed pitted olives
6 large sun-dried tomatoes
2 large handfuls of basil
3–4 handfuls of rocket leaves
2–3 tablespoons white wine vinegar
Sea salt

Makes 4 large portions

TOPPER pictured

1 Steam the cauliflower for 2–3 minutes until al dente.
2 Add the flat 'chopper' blade to the top of the food processor. Replace the lid. Place the celery into the opening at the top while turning the food processor on. Push it through with the added attachment until flatly finely sliced. Once chopped, place into a waiting bowl.
3 Next, change the blades over so the central chopping attachment is in place. Add the cauliflower and pulse until it forms chunky and even chopped pieces.
4 Repeat the above with the mangetout, olives and sun-dried tomatoes. The tomatoes and olives will go into a paste. Stir into the mix.
5 Roughly hand-chop the basil and rocket and mix into the veg.
6 Drizzle with white wine vinegar and sprinkle with sea salt.

toppers

Pistachio nuts add a nice decorative creamy, but crunchy TOPPER.

morph your slaw
Provence Scramble

1 Mix any leftover slaw into 3 whisked eggs.
2 Pan-fry gently until the egg is cooked into a scramble, about 5 minutes.

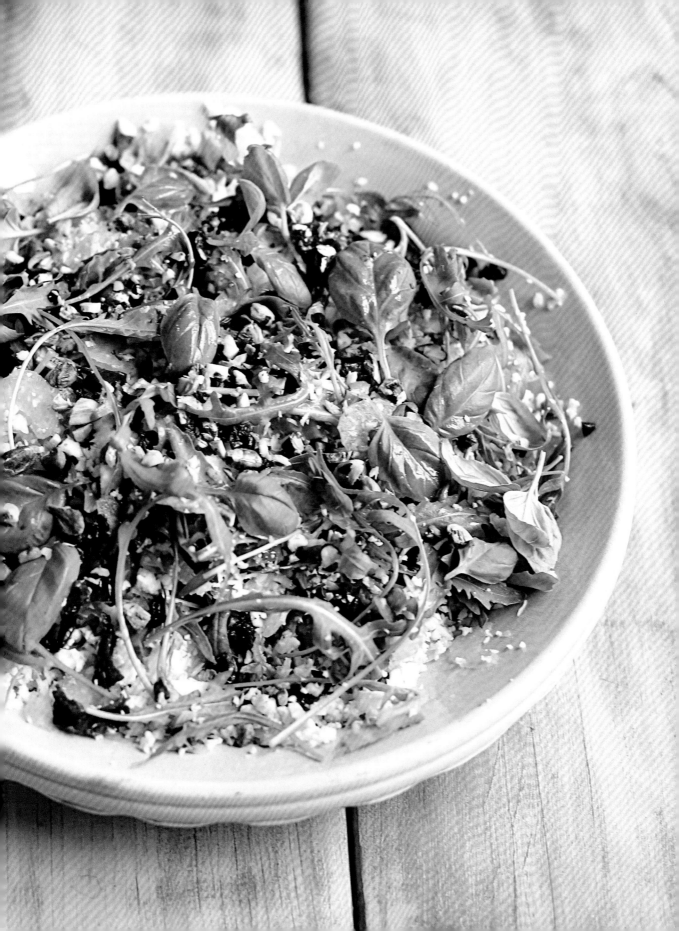

Coco-Lime Slaw

The benefits of the coconut craze seem to be holding their own in the food market as coconut has a unique fat content and antibacterial properties, perfect for keeping the skin glowing!

My method for coconut extraction is to use a corkscrew at the eye (the softest of the three indentations at the base) to drain or drink the water. You can now tell how fresh it is (off coconut has a pungent odour). Wrap in a plastic bag, take it outside and, holding firmly, hit it on the ground to break in half. Use a knife to separate the flesh from the shell.

2–3 handfuls of coconut pieces
¼ medium white cabbage, core removed
6 stalks of celery
¼ red onion
1 large red chilli, deseeded
2–3 limes, halved
Sea salt

Makes 4 large portions

MORPH pictured

1 Place the central chopping attachment in the main bowl of the food processor, followed by the coconut pieces and replace the lid. Pulse on the highest setting (due to the density of the coconut) until chopped into very fine pieces. Keep your hand firmly on the lid. Alternatively, you can grate the coconut if you struggle to chop this in the food processor. Tip the coconut into a waiting bowl.

2 Repeat the above on a lower setting with the cabbage and celery stalks (aim for a more chunky chop) and mix in the bowl with the coconut.

3 Hand-slice the red onion and chilli into small, even pieces and mix in.

4 Squeeze with the juice of the limes and sprinkle with the sea salt.

toppers

Macadamia nuts and cucumber pieces make delicious TOPPERS for extra good fats and hydration.

morph your slaw
Coco-Lime-Coco Soup

1 Boil a 400ml tin of coconut milk in a pan with a little extra vegetable or chicken stock.

2 Add some lemongrass and ginger pieces.

3 Add in any leftover slaw and simmer for 5–6 minutes.

4 Remove the lemongrass.

5 Add in chicken slices and noodles and cook through, about 12 minutes.

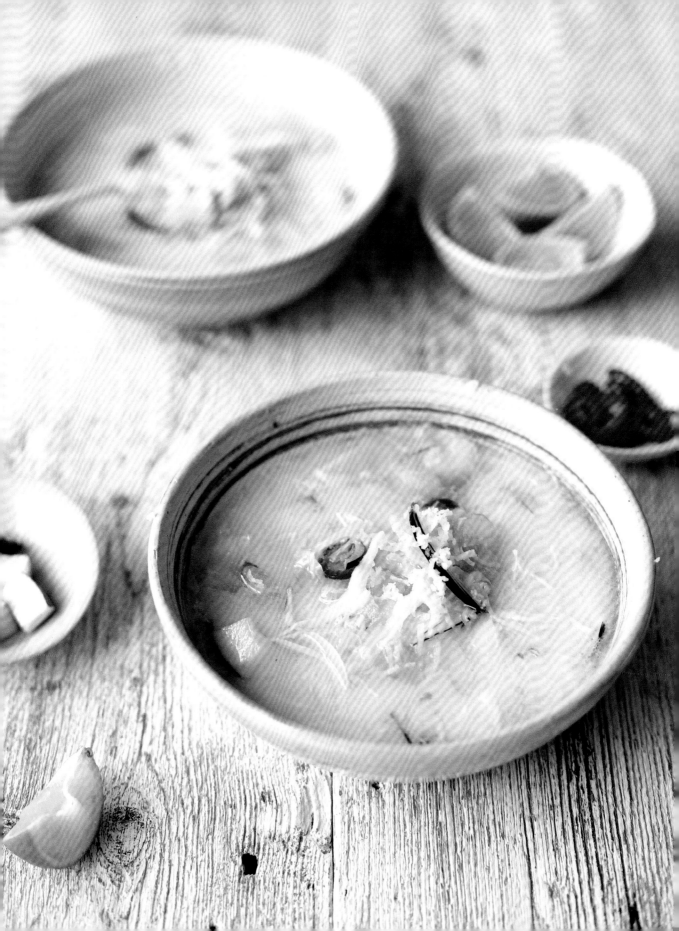

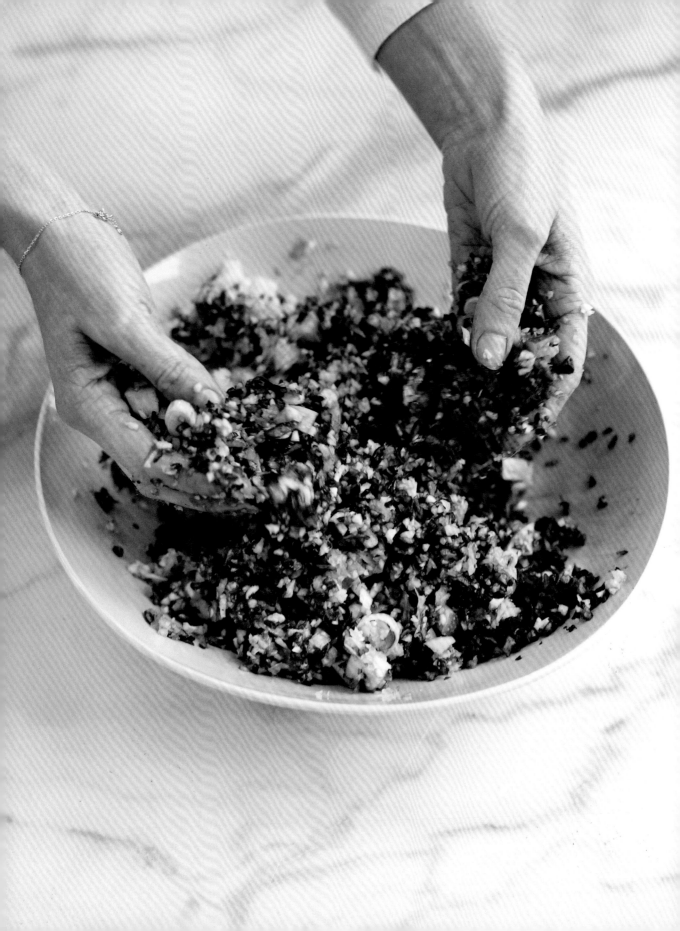

Celeriac Slaw

Celeriac (also known as knob celery) is not the most attractive of root vegetables so it is understandable why it is often overlooked. However, the crunchiness of this particular veg, added to the useful vitamin content and the fact it is super-low in calories, makes it a powerful slaw base. With a similar taste to celery, but with a heavier and slightly nutty flavour, it works well with the sweetness of an apple. Cooked celeriac makes a lighter alternative to mash – check out the slaw MORPH for an even more exciting version of a chunky slaw mash served with a rich fatty fish such as salmon.

1 medium celeriac, peeled and chopped into chunky pieces
1 small red cabbage, core removed and chopped into quarters
4 stalks of celery
2 green chillies, deseeded
2 apples (any sweet variety), cored
2–3 tablespoons cider vinegar
2–3 tablespoons olive oil
Sea salt

Makes 4 large portions

1 Place the central chopping attachment into the main bowl of the food processor.

2 Add the celeriac to the main bowl of the food processor and pulse until it forms chunky pieces. Celeriac is a tough, fibrous veg, so this will be a noisy blitz! Keep your hand firmly on the lid. Add to a waiting bowl

3 Repeat the chop with the red cabbage, then the celery, and add all into the bowl together.

4 Slice the chillies and apples into very fine pieces, then add to the vegetables and mix well.

5 Add the vinegar and olive oil to a jam jar. Place the lid on and shake vigorously. Add to the slaw.

6 Season with a sprinkle of sea salt and mix together well.

toppers

Avocado and a sprinkle of pumpkin seeds boosts the vitamin B-complex and adds good-quality fats.

morph your slaw
Chunky Celeriac Mash with Salmon

1 Boil some celeriac for 10–15 minutes in a pan until soft enough to mash.

2 Mix in any leftover slaw to create a chunky, crunchy mash.

3 Serve with some grilled salmon.

Pizza Slaw

Who would have thought that pizza could be good for your skin? If you follow the Topper tip for this slaw you can achieve the flavour of pizza, but without maxing your calorie quota for the day. Research shows that tomatoes help protect against sunburn and skin ageing caused by the effects of UV exposure. This is all down to the antioxidant lycopene (which gives tomatoes their red colour). It is most effective when heated.

2 courgettes
1 large tub (around 250 g) of
*   mini tomatoes*
1 red onion
½ red chilli, deseeded
1 garlic clove
1 tablespoon dried oregano
1–2 tablespoons tomato purée
3–4 tablespoons red wine vinegar
Sea salt

Makes 4 large portions

1 Place the courgette in a food processor and pulse the button until chopped. Remove any extra chunky pieces and pop back in if you need to (courgette is a tricky customer for a consistent chop!). Place in a waiting bowl.

2 Repeat with the tomatoes. They will blitz in seconds, so avoid over-pulsing.

3 Hand-chop the onion, chilli and garlic into thin slices and add to the mix.

4 Sprinkle with oregano and mix.

5 Squeeze the tomato purée over the mix and add the vinegar. Depending how the mixture stirs, you may need to add a little extra vinegar.

6 Mix well and sprinkle with sea salt.

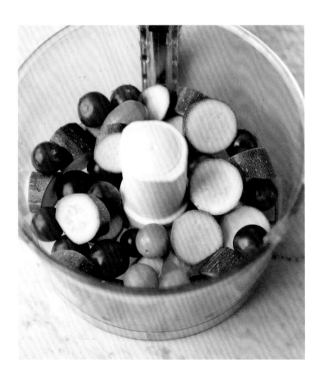

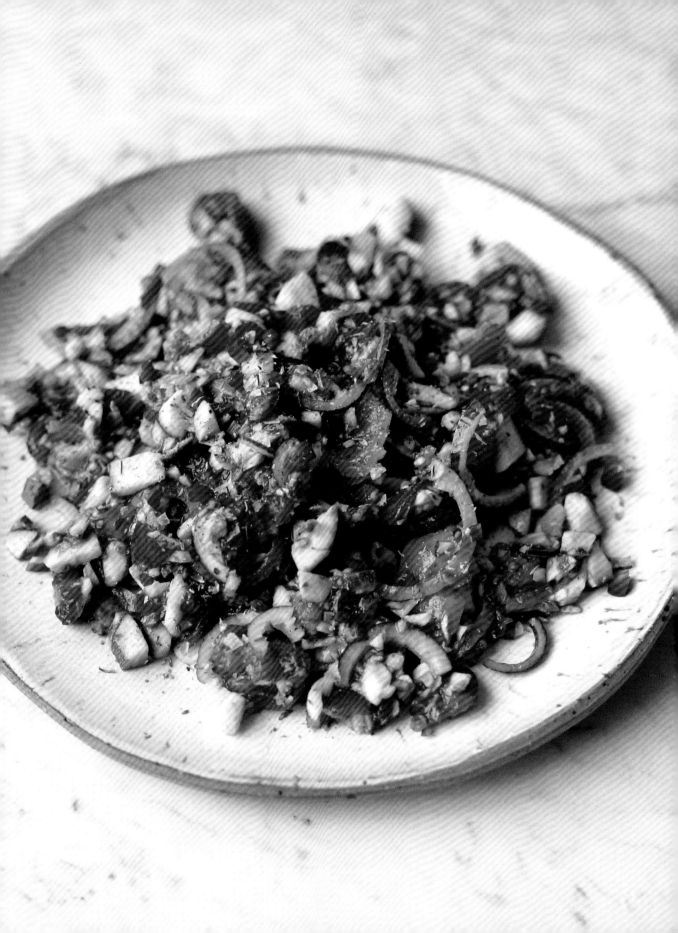

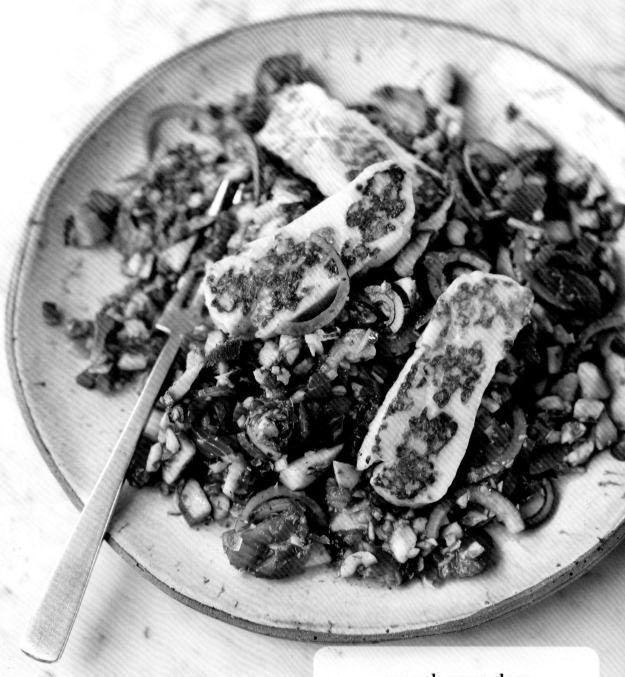

toppers

Halloumi is great with this slaw, though mozzarella is perhaps a more obvious (and a slightly lower calorie) choice for a traditional pizza flavour.

morph your slaw

Pizza Wrap

1 Place any left over slaw in a flatbread.

2 Add in a few slices of grilled cheese.

3 Add a little chopped and fried chorizo sausage and some freshly steamed kale.

4 Roll into a burrito shape and serve straightaway.

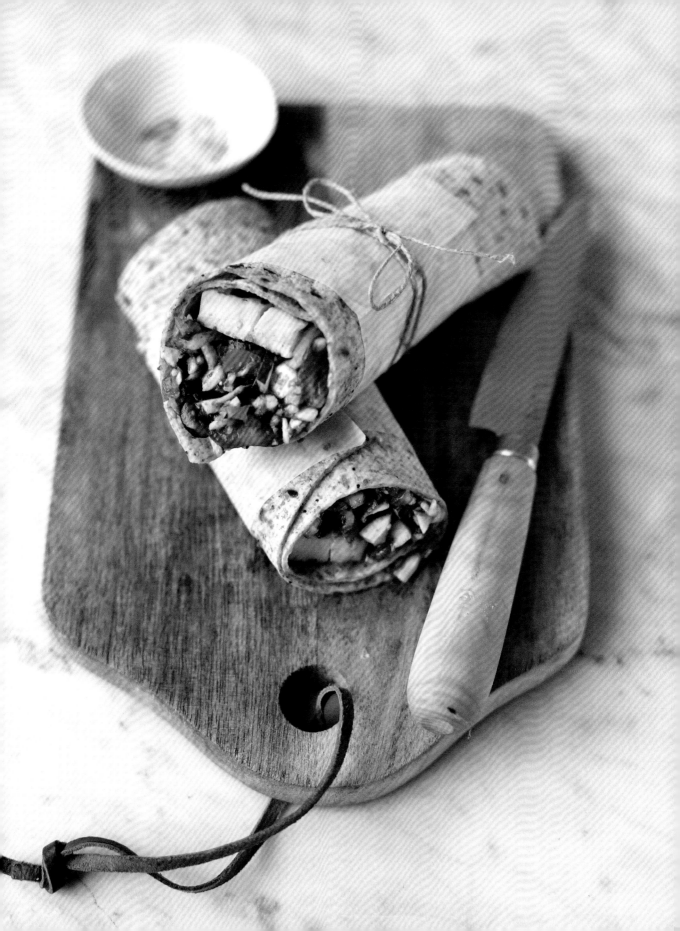

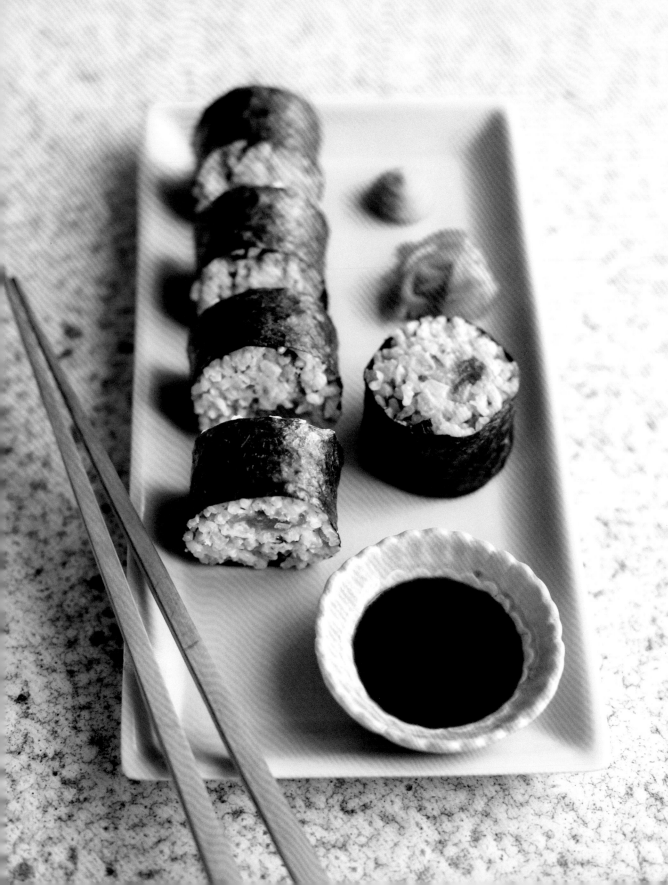

Tzatziki Slaw

Tzatziki Slaw is a super way of adding an influx of instant hydration in to a meal. Supplying anti-aging vitamins like C and carotenes (vitamin A), cucumbers are also a source of silica, the trace mineral that contributes to skin health by aiding reproduction of connective tissue. The skin of the cucumber is known to hold just as many benefits as the flesh, so try and go for organic where possible.

This is best eaten close to preparation time. If using the processor, the trick is to click the button instantaneously on and off four to five times.

2 large cucumbers, cut into quarters
1 handful of green olives, pitted
2 garlic cloves
½ green chilli, deseeded
1 small pot (150 g) of natural yoghurt (go for full-fat where possible)
1 tablespoon white wine vinegar
Sea salt

Makes 4 large portions

MORPH pictured

1 Place the cucumbers in a food processor and 'click' the button four to five times until the cucumber is chopped into chunks (erring on the side of caution with the button). Add the cucumber to a sieve and drain away any excess water before popping into a bowl.

2 Chop the olives, garlic and chilli (although this is super easy to do by hand, I love the paste it helps create by adding to the food processor). Mix in with the cucumber.

3 Mix the full pot of yoghurt with the vinegar.

4 Mix well and season generously with sea salt.

toppers

Seaweed flakes (nori) are a favourite crispy TOPPER. They provide a lovely crispy, salty flavour. Crunch up and sprinkle onto the slaw.

morph your slaw
Nori Tzatziki Slaw Wrap

1 Layer a nori (seaweed sheet) with some pre-cooked warm rice.

2 Add any leftover slaw and spread out.

3 Layer with cooked cold seafood, such as smoked salmon, and roll into a delicious wrap.

Papaya Slaw

Papaya reminds me of my visits to Thailand. It's the perfect complement to a spicy red chilli, and famed for its digestive benefits. For this slaw, make sure you choose a papaya that is fully green and really firm when you press it. If you can't find papaya, you can replace it with pieces of peeled cucumber or melon (sliced by hand), which are also reported to be great for digestion. Papaya can go slimy if left too long, so serve immediately.

2 green papaya
2 limes, halved
½ teaspoon sugar or a drizzle of honey (optional), to sweeten
2 handfuls of parsley, roughly chopped
1 red chilli, deseeded and roughly chopped
3 spring onions, roughly chopped
Handful of crushed brazil nuts (cashews work well too)
Drizzle of olive oil
1 handful of poppy seeds
Sea salt

Makes 4 large portions

1 Peel the papaya and slice in half. Scoop any seeds or pith from the centre. Use a mandolin or grater to chop the papaya into thin strips. You can also use a peeler for this.
2 Place in a bowl and squeeze the lime and optional sugar or honey over it.
3 Add the parsley, chilli and spring onions to the papaya.
4 Add the crushed nuts.
5 Drizzle with olive oil and sprinkle with poppy seeds and sea salt.

toppers

Dried shrimps, found in many Asian stores, make a great TOPPER for this dish's gentle flavours. Alternatively, opt for other seafood, such as fresh prawns or crayfish.

morph your slaw
Papaya Prawn Stir-fry

1 Heat a few drops of fish sauce in a pan.
2 Stir-fry prawns until pink, about 2–3 minutes.
3 Add in any leftover slaw, cook for a further 1–2 minutes and serve.

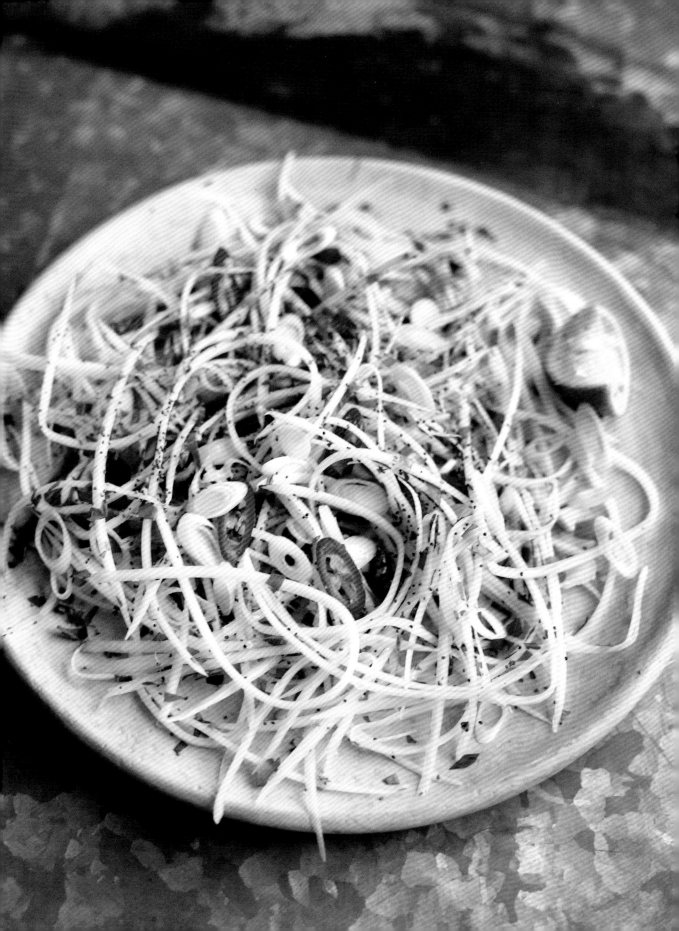

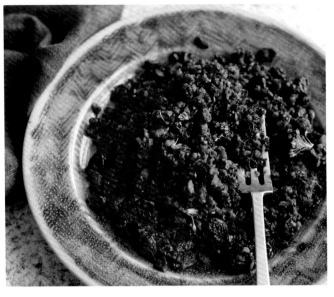

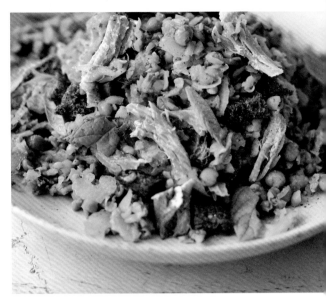

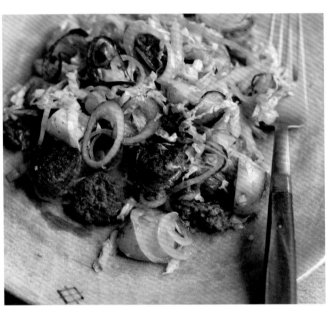

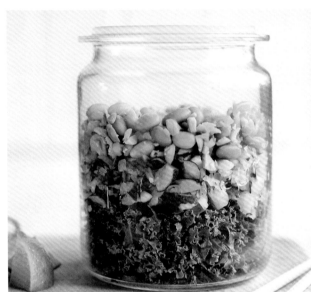

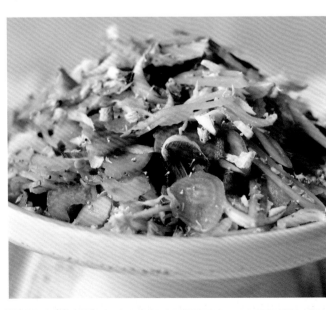

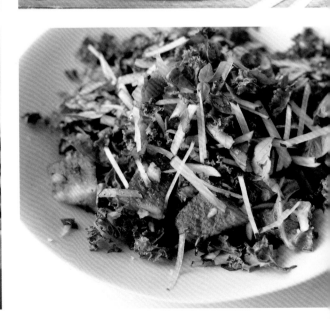

Recovery

Need to recover from a long hike in the hills or a tough session in the gym? Look no further than the Recovery SuperSlaw. I created these recipes when I noticed certain food cravings on workout days. I did a little research into the things I had been hankering after and I soon found commonalties amongst many of the ingredients, which appeared to play a beneficial part in post-workout recovery.

Recent research has pointed to the benefits of beetroot and vinegar in helping recovery and endurance. These recipes are perfect for people who exercise regularly and want to test the theory behind the beetroot blast! If you're not a beetroot fan, you can swap it for other veggies with higher carbohydrate stores, such as root vegetables, but you may want to cook them first to ease digestion.

When training continuously or at high levels of intensity, glycogen (the storage form of carbohydrate found in the liver and muscles) is depleted, so it makes sense to keep the meals you eat on 'training days' higher in carbohydrate. Don't forget the importance of protein and adequate hydration in this process, which are also pivotal in the process of rebuilding muscle tissue. Recovery SuperSlaws are all recommended to be eaten with a good protein source, and can be topped up with extra carbohydrates if you know you have had a particularly challenging day of training.

The main focus after any period of intense exercise should be to help the body both replenish any lost fuel and repair any damage caused. This will aid energy stores to be renewed, and an overall improved recovery. Antioxidant-rich foods will also benefit the immune system, which is put through its paces at periods of intensity!

Add a little extra sea salt after super-hot and sweaty sessions to help counterbalance any lost electrolytes that were left on your gym towel!

Pea + Mint Slaw

Peas are loaded with vitamins and minerals and this slaw also looks pretty impressive on a table, making it one of my most popular requests. Don't worry about using frozen peas; just slightly defrost them by running through cold water in a sieve for up to a minute. By the time you put them through the food processor they will be thawed enough to eat. Using frozen peas will also keep it from becoming too mushy and will last longer.

1 bag (150 g) of sugar snap peas
6–8 stalks of celery stalks, cut into quarters
½ jar (150–200 g) gherkins or cornichons, drained from any vinegar
1 small bag (200 g) of frozen peas, slightly defrosted by placing in cold water, then draining
3 tablespoons mint sauce
2–4 tablespoons white wine vinegar
Black pepper
Fresh and/or dried mint, to garnish (optional)

Makes 4 large portions

TOPPER pictured

1 Place the central chopping attachment into the main bowl of the food processor.
2 Place the sugar snaps, celery and gherkins in the main bowl. Pulse until evenly chopped (you may have to do this in batches). Place in a waiting bowl.
3 Repeat with the peas until they are slightly chopped, but not mushy. Add to the other vegetables.
4 Add the mint sauce and vinegar to a jam jar. Place the lid on and shake vigorously. Pour over the slaw and mix well. Season with black pepper to taste.
5 Garnish with fresh and/or dried mint (optional).

toppers

Pea mint and ham hock make a beautiful salad. Top with ham hock pieces and some home-toasted rye bread croutons for a full macronutrient meal.

morph your slaw
Pea + Mint Soup

1 Sauté some white onion in a pan with a little oil.
2 Add a couple of cups of vegetable or chicken stock and bring to the boil.
3 Roughly chop a handful of new potatoes and add them to the pan. Gently boil until the potatoes are cooked through, about 10 minutes.
4 Add any leftover slaw, top with a knob of butter or a drop of cream, remove from the heat and blitz in a blender until liquidised. Serve hot or cold.

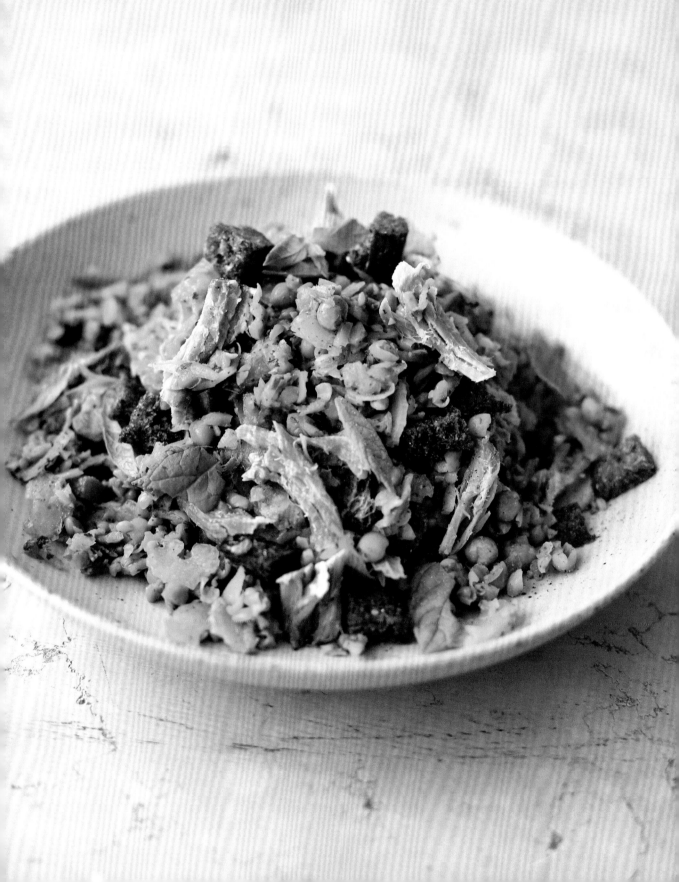

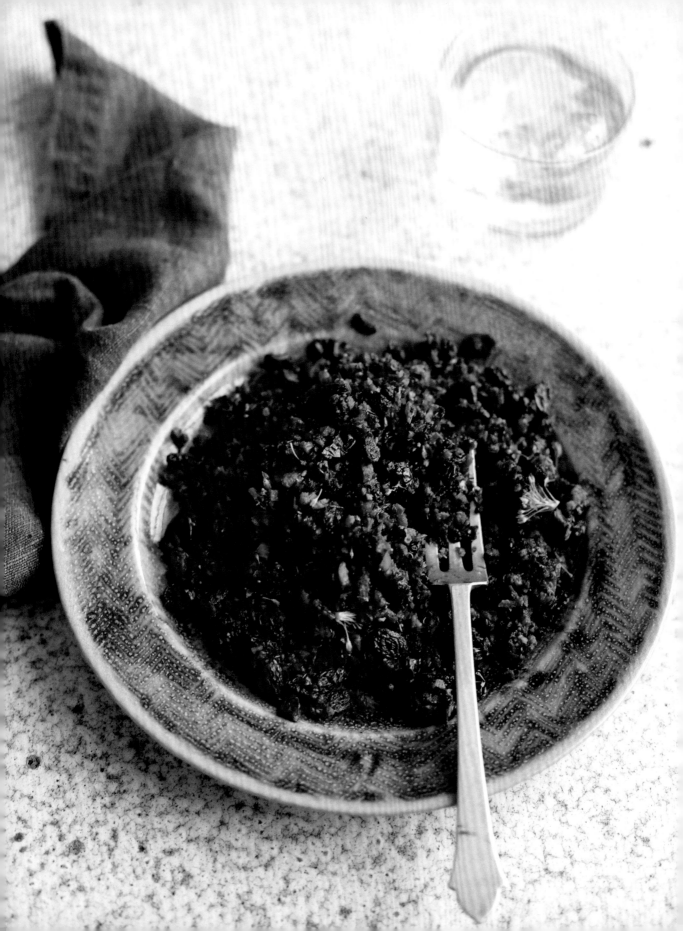

Purple Punch Slaw

I embrace the colour purple in both food and life. I can't think of any natural purple foods that I don't love the flavour of, and food experts believe purple vegetables top the chart for health benefits. Purple foods contain anthocyanins, a type of pigment that is powerful in antioxidants, protecting cells from damage, slowing down blood clotting and with anti-ageing benefits! The dried fruits in this slaw are the prefect sugary addition for following a particularly tough workout. MORPH your slaw for a full, rounded macronutrient meal.

2 large handfuls of purple
   sprouting broccoli
1 packet (250–300 g) of
   cooked beetroot
6 medium carrots, peeled
2 small handfuls of mixed raisins/
   sultanas
1 small handful of dried cranberries
1–2 tablespoons balsamic vinegar
1–2 tablespoons white balsamic
   vinegar
1 tablespoon olive oil
Sea salt

Makes 4 large portions

1 Place the central chopping attachment into the main bowl of the food processor and add the broccoli to the cooked beetroot. Pulse very gently until chopped. The beetroot will coat the broccoli.

2 Repeat with the carrots. As a dense vegetable they will take a little extra 'pulsing'. Once chopped, add to the mix.

3 Sprinkle the mixture with the dried fruits and stir well.

4 Put the vinegars, olive oil and a sprinkle of sea salt into a jam jar. Fix on the lid and shake vigorously.

5 Pour over the slaw and mix well.

toppers

For an extra crunchy antioxidant boost, top this slaw with some chopped up yellow pepper.

morph your slaw

Purple Punch Couscous Salad with Chicken

1 Cook some couscous according to the packet instructions.

2 Mix with any leftover slaw.

3 Top with a grilled chicken breast.

Tutti-Frutti Slaw

Ginger holds anti-inflammatory benefits, which are said to be so strong
that some studies show it helps reduce post-exercise workout pain.
This Tutti-Frutti mix is a little like a savoury fruit salad, with a bit more
gumption! Tutti-Frutti helps to rehydrate the body, with some super-fast
antioxidants. It works as a starter, main course or even a great snack, with
salty flavours such as smoky bacon or ham.

1 apple
1 pear
1 small white cabbage, core
   removed and chopped into
   quarters
½ packet (175 g) of cooked
   beetroot
1 pomegranate, deseeded or 2
   packets (100 g) of pomegranate
   seeds (see page 30)
2–3 tablespoons balsamic vinegar
Squeeze of ½ lemon or lime
1 cm cube of fresh ginger, peeled
   and grated
Sea salt
Blueberries, to garnish

Makes 4 large portions

1 Place the apple, pear and cabbage into the main bowl of the food
   processor, with the central chopping attachment. Pulse until chunkily
   chopped and add to a waiting bowl.

2 Repeat with the beetroot and add to the mix.

3 Stir the ingredients well and sprinkle with pomegranate seeds.

4 Drizzle with the vinegar. Squeeze in the lemon or lime.

5 Mix in the grated ginger and sprinkle with sea salt.

6 Garnish the slaw with blueberries and serve.

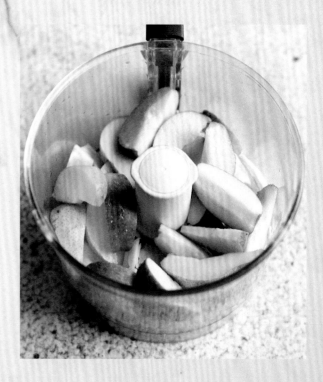

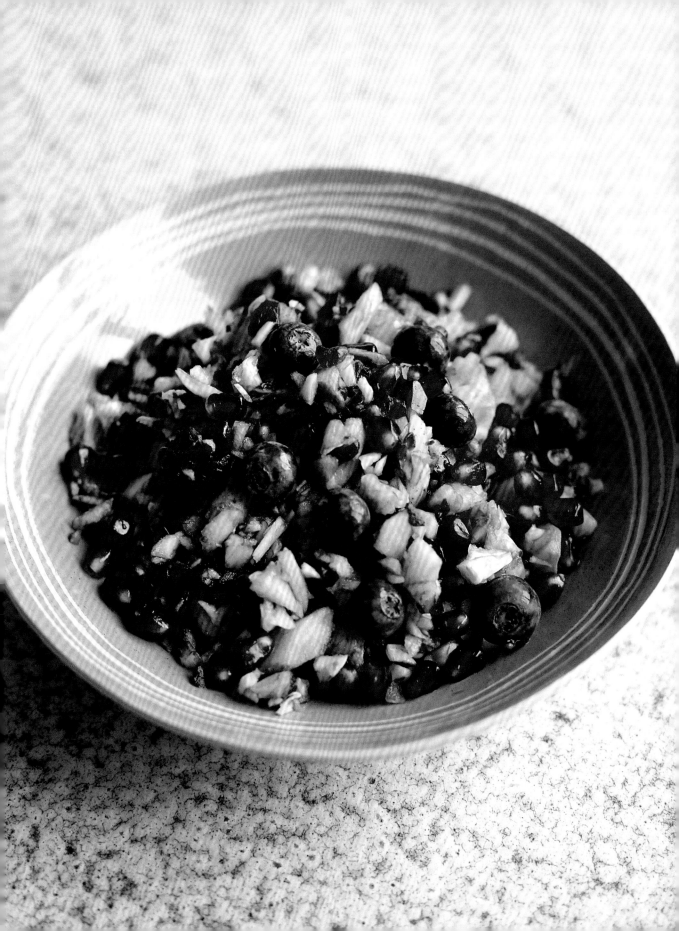

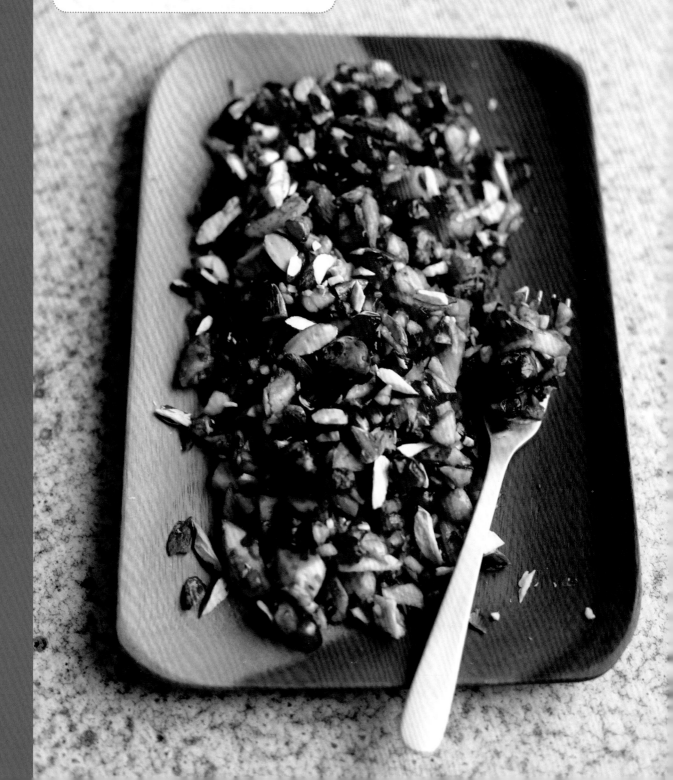

toppers

A small handful of crushed salted almonds works
perfectly as a crunchy TOPPER.

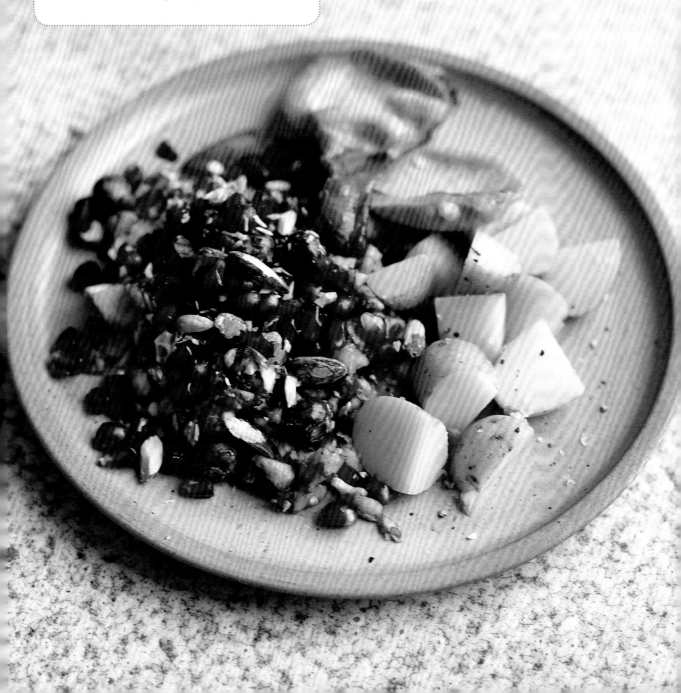

morph your slaw
Tutti-Frutti Bacon Salad

1 Boil some new potatoes until cooked, about 10 minutes.

2 Grill some lean pieces of bacon for a few minutes on each side.

3 Serve the bacon and potatoes with the slaw.

Japanese Edamame Slaw

Adding good-quality but diverse, lean protein sources to a post-workout meal can be difficult to achieve sometimes so I wanted to try and utilize some alternative items that have become more convenient to buy on supermarket shelves. The Japanese edamame bean contains a complete profile of amino acids, the building blocks of muscle repair. Top with a touch of ginger for extra anti-inflammatory benefits and feel the hydrating benefits from the radish to refill those water stores, making this a winning SuperSlaw for after a heavy, sweaty session in the gym.

250 g radishes, topped and tailed
200 g edamame beans (I buy the
* pre-cooked and podded beans)*
100 g kale
1 lime, halved
2 tablespoons white miso paste
1 tablespoon rice wine vinegar
1 tablespoon soy sauce (I use
* reduced-sodium)*
1 tablespoon sesame oil
2 tablespoons olive oil

Makes 4 large portions

1 Place the radishes into the main bowl of the food processor with the central chopping attachment and pulse gently until cut into even chunks. Place in a waiting bowl.

2 Add the edamame beans and kale and repeat (try to ensure the beans don't go too mushy). Add to the radish pieces.

3 Squeeze the lime over the mixture.

4 Pour the miso, along with the vinegar, soy sauce and oils into an empty jam jar. Shake vigorously until mixed.

5 Pour over the vegetables and mix well.

toppers

Top with grated fresh ginger and spring onion.

morph your slaw
Japanese Layered Rice Salad

1 Boil Japanese sushi rice until light and fluffy following the packet instructions. Allow to cool.

2 Layer rice in the bottom of a bowl.

3 Layer any leftover slaw on top of the rice.

4 Sprinkle with your choice of steamed fish.

5 Garnish with a sprinkle of spring onion.

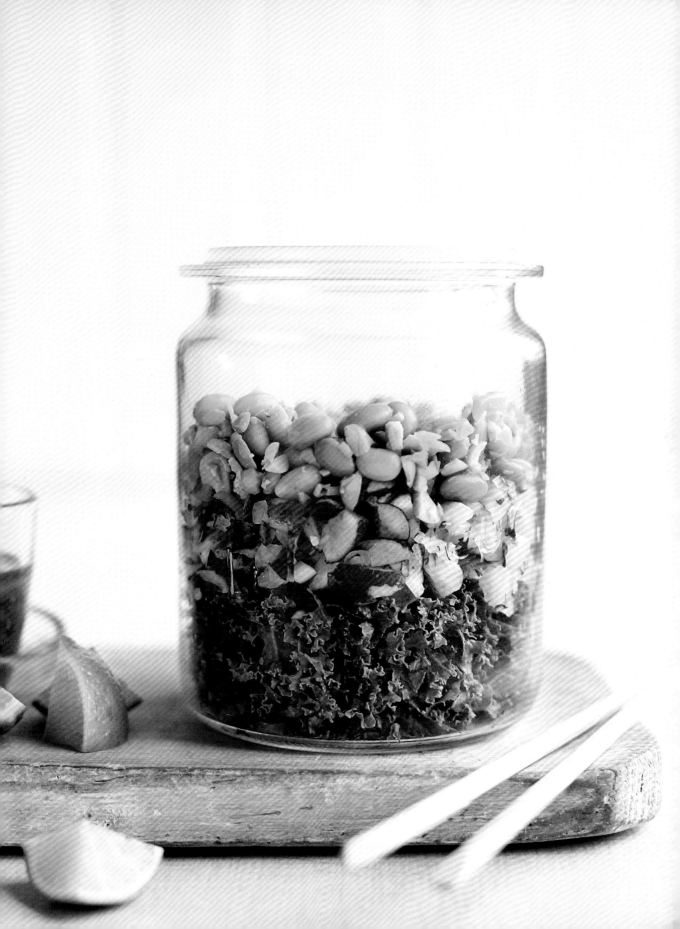

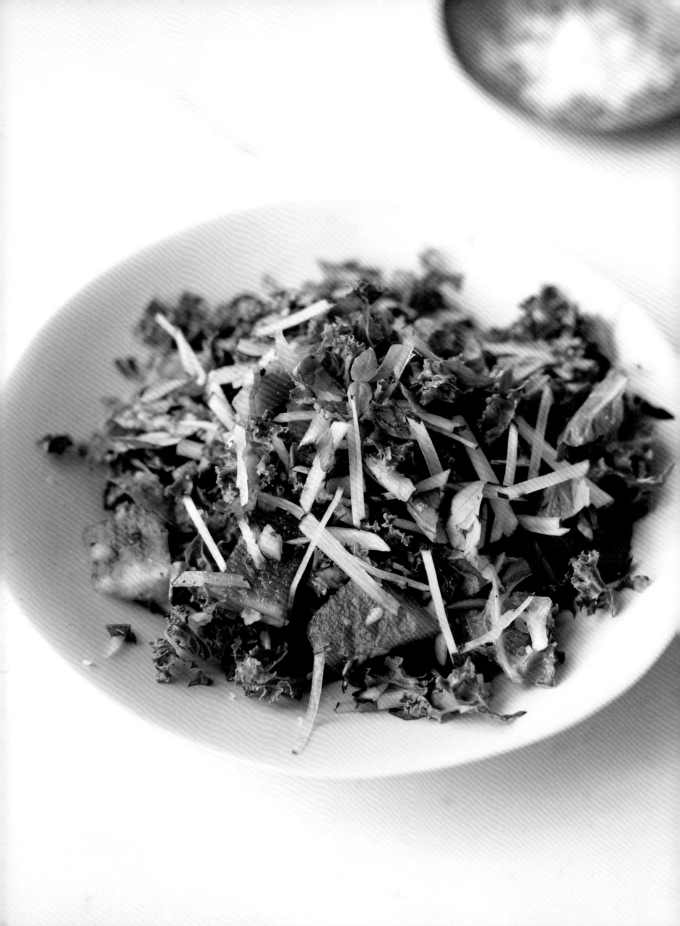

Watermelon + Basil Slaw

Unsurprisingly, watermelon is high in water, but it also contains heaps of vitamins, and some potassium and magnesium too, making it a fantastic natural electrolyte. Electrolytes are ionic solutions that keep your body, muscle and nerves functioning properly.

Watermelon is believed to contain the amino acid citrulline. In fact the name itself is said to be derived from the Latin word citrullus, which actually means watermelon! Citrulline contributes multiple benefits for the body, most notably an increase in blood flow, which is perfect for aiding the process of post-workout recovery.

200 g radishes, topped and tailed
4 large handfuls of kale
½ red onion
2 large handfuls of basil
2 large handfuls of mint
1 small cube of fresh ginger, peeled
Drizzle of olive oil
200 g cubed watermelon
Sea salt

Makes 4 large portions

1 Place the radishes and kale into the main bowl of the food processor with the central chopping attachment. Pulse until chunkily chopped. Pour into a waiting bowl.
2 Repeat with the onion and herbs, then add to the mix.
3 Grate the ginger over the vegetables (or you can hand-chop into tiny pieces) and stir in.
4 Mix the ingredients together and drizzle with olive oil until coated.
5 Mix in the watermelon pieces.
6 Season with sea salt.

toppers
Top with Parma ham pieces and cottage cheese for a protein kick.

morph your slaw
Parma Ham Stuffed Watermelon Rolls

1 Place torn strips of Parma ham on a flat surface.
2 Cook some sticky rice according to packet instructions and allow to cool.
3 Mix any leftover slaw with the rice.
4 Layer the mixture onto the Parma ham pieces and roll into small sausage shapes.

Beetroot Blast Slaw

This is a real overload of beetroot, so perfect if you have had a particularly hard workout. It is also super-quick to make, so ideal for anyone in a hurry to eat or suffering with post-workout hunger.

It makes a great snack when mixing a few spoonfuls into mashed smoked fish such as mackerel. In the food processor, cooked beetroot is just dense enough to hold a good consistency, while also mashing a little, creating a lovely sweet coating for the veggies. The horseradish then gives a nice little kick to help balance the sugary flavour.

1 packet (250 g) of cooked beetroot
1 bag (150 g) of mangetout
4 large handfuls of rocket leaves
2–3 tablespoons balsamic vinegar
1 tablespoon horseradish sauce
Sea salt

Makes 4 large portions

1 Place the central chopping attachment into the main bowl of the food processor.
2 Place the beetroot into the main bowl along with the mangetout and rocket leaves. Pulse until finely chopped.
3 Pour the vinegar into a jam jar with the horseradish and a sprinkle of salt. Replace the lid and shake well. Pour over the slaw and mix well.

toppers

Pan-fried, peeled sweet potato shavings will add an extra starchy carbohydrate boost.

morph your slaw

Smoked Mackerel Beetroot Blast

1 Flake peppered smoked mackerel into a bowl.
2 Mix in any leftover slaw and stir together.
3 Serve on a rice or oat cake.

Courgette, Tomato + Quark Slaw

Quark should be in every workout lover's secret fitness recipe kit. High in protein, low in fat and a lot less calories than many alternative soft cheeses, quark is perfect to help the body recover by providing 'casein', a high-quality and slow-release protein, ensuring more prolonged support for muscle growth.

3 courgettes
½ white onion
1 small handful of sun-dried
  tomatoes
2 heaped tablespoons quark
3–4 tablespoons white wine vinegar
Sea salt

Makes 4 large portions

1 Place the courgettes into the main bowl of the food processor with the central chopping attachment and pulse gently until cut into even chunks. Courgette is high in water, so try and avoid over-pulsing. Place in a waiting bowl.

2 Add the onion and sun-dried tomatoes to the main bowl of the food processor and repeat. The mixture will be a little like a chunky paste. Add to an empty jam jar.

3 Spoon the quark, vinegar and a sprinkle of sea salt into the jar with the onion and tomato paste.

4 Shake vigorously until mixed. Add a little more vinegar if the mixture is too thick.

5 Pour over the courgette and mix well.

toppers

Top with mixed beans for a carbohydrate source.

morph your slaw

Stuffed Potato Skins

1 Bake 2 large sweet potatoes in a 200°C oven until soft, about 50 minutes.

2 Allow to cool and cut in half, spoon out the soft potato mix and mash.

3 Mix the mash into any leftover slaw and place back into the skins.

4 Grill until cooked through.

Baby Potato + Red Spring Onion Slaw

The humble spud has been neglected in recent low-carb years, which is a great shame for a food that is not only incredibly beneficial for health, but also readily available. Potatoes are a high carbohydrate food, which is ideal for aiding the body restore depleted glycogen (meaning less chance of muscle stiffness and more chance of lean muscle growth).

Red onions are one of the best natural sources of quercetin, a bioflavonoid that helps scavenge free radicals.

1 whole Chinese leaf cabbage, cut into quarters
2 large red spring onions
1 lemon, halved
Dash of Worcestershire sauce
1 teaspoon French mustard
Sea salt
Drizzle of olive oil
3–4 handfuls of cooked baby new potatoes, allowed to cool

Makes 4 large portions

MORPH pictured

1 Place the Chinese leaf into the main bowl of the food processor with the central chopping attachment and pulse gently until cut into even strips. Place into a waiting bowl.
2 Hand-chop the red spring onions into fine slices and mix in with the Chinese leaf.
3 Squeeze the juice of the lemon into an empty jam jar. Add the Worcestershire sauce, French mustard, salt and a dash of olive oil. Shake vigorously until mixed.
4 Pour over the vegetables and mix well.
5 Mix into the cooked potatoes.

toppers

Add pre-cooked prawns for a lean source of protein.

morph your slaw

Hot Chorizo + Baby Potato Slaw

1 Pan-fry chopped pieces of cooked chorizo in a heavy-based frying pan. Heat until the fat of the sausage drizzles into the pan. Remove the sausage and set aside.
2 Pour any leftover slaw into the pan and heat through. Coat the mixture with the pan oil.
3 Add the chorizo back in and serve.

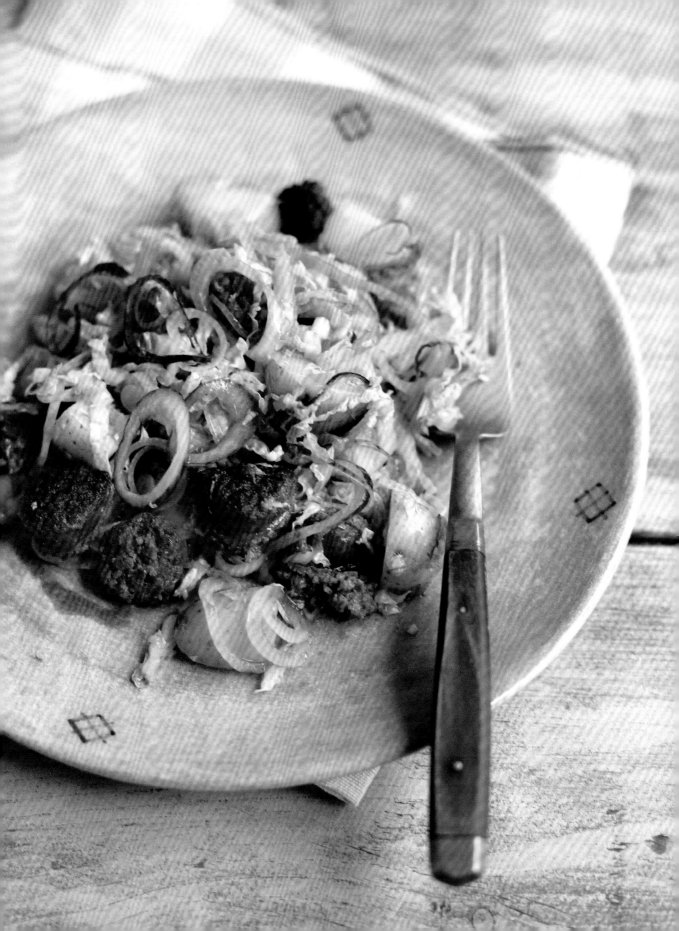

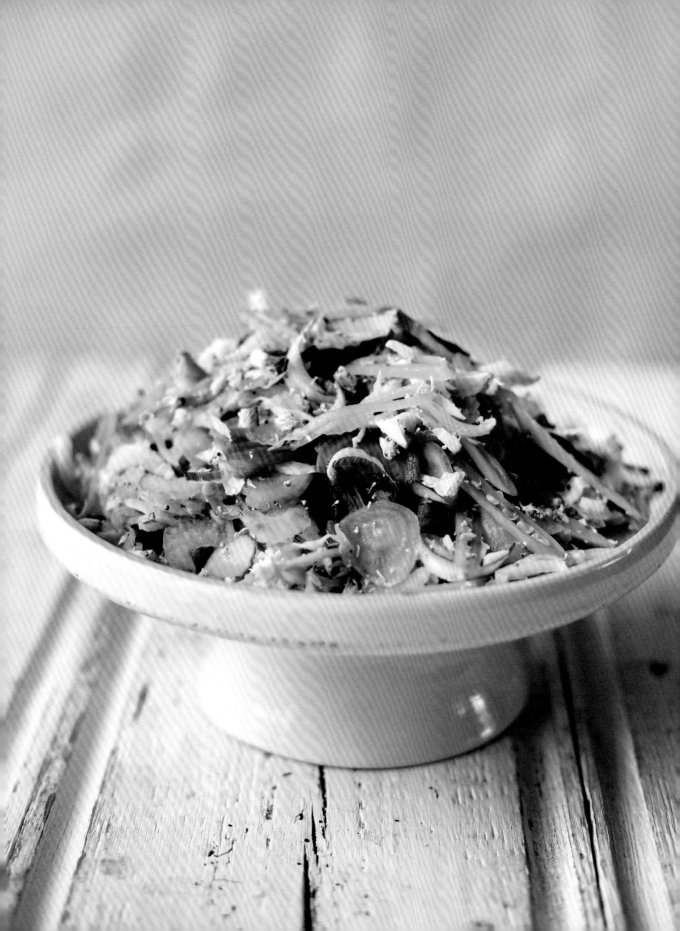

Sweet + Sour Apple Slaw

When I first suggested the idea of apple sauce mixed with gherkins my partner thought I'd gone crazy! But when he tried it he loved it. The sweet and sour flavours complement each other so well.

   I find that apple sauce is an often forgotten condiment in the fridge that could do with a little help getting used, and this is a great recipe for it. My Nan was a big advocate of using what you already have to make good food so I'm dedicating this one to her.

1 head (400g) of broccoli
2 heads of chicory, sliced
1 bag (150 g) of sugar snap peas
8 large gherkins
1 packet (250–300 g) of cooked
   beetroot
6 stalks of celery
3 tablespoons white wine vinegar
1 tablespoon apple sauce
Sea salt

Makes 4 large portions

1 Place the central chopping attachment into the main bowl of the food processor, followed by the broccoli and then replace the lid.
2 Pulse the broccoli to a chunky-chopped texture before tipping into a waiting bowl.
3 Repeat with the chicory heads and sugar snaps peas (they will take less time to chop) and add these to the chopped broccoli.
4 Put the gherkins and beetroot into the mixer and pulse (beware, this will literally take a second). Tip over the chopped vegetables.
5 Change attachments, using the flat 'chopper' blade to chop the celery, and then pour into the mix.
6 Put the vinegar and apple sauce into a jam jar. Fix on the lid and shake vigorously.
7 Pour over the slaw and mix.
8 Season with sea salt.

toppers

For a perfect post-workout combo, add a good-quality protein source such as soft-boiled runny eggs.

morph your slaw

Minced Sweet + Spicy Turkey Fry

1 Pan-fry minced turkey in a dash of coconut oil until cooked, about 6–7 minutes.
2 Sprinkle with dried chilli.
3 Add in the slaw and pan-fry for 1–2 minutes.
4 Serve with boiled basmati rice or quinoa.

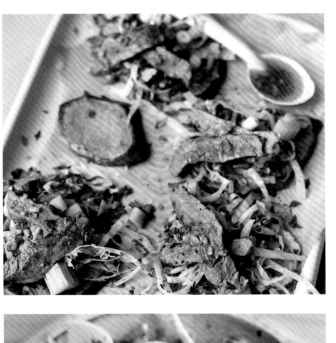

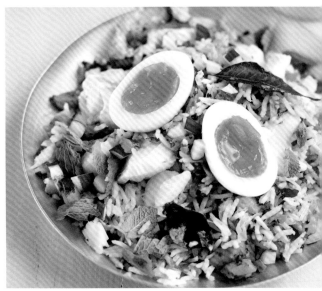

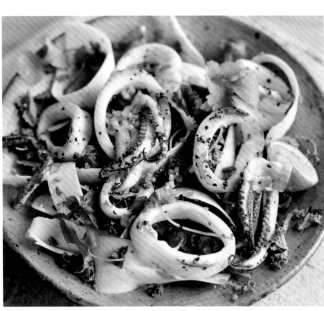

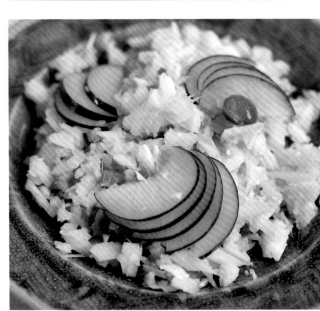

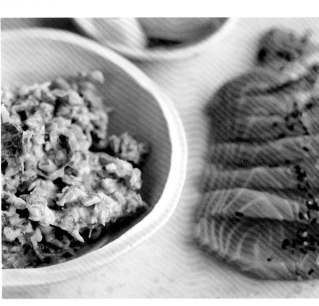

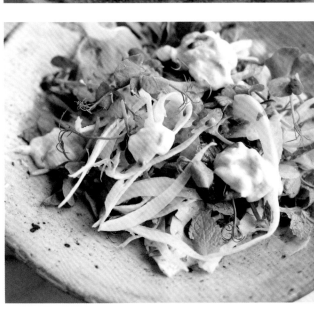

Thermic + Spicy

All foods are known to have an almost stimulatory impact on the body, known as the 'thermic effect'. This describes the metabolic process set off to expend energy for activities such as digestion, and the absorption, transportation or elimination of food nutrients to the cells of your body.

Not all foods are processed equally by the body and research suggests that some foods have a greater 'thermic influence' than others. Protein, for example, has a greater thermic effect than carbohydrate, and carbohydrate more so than fat. Whilst the science in this area is ongoing, there is an overwhelming agreement that foods such as green tea, caffeine and chillies (capsaicin, see below) have been proven to have an almost metabolic booster effect on the body.

My Thermic Spicy SuperSlaws are just the ticket for working with this principle of using heat for those sneaky extra benefits. I have converted many reluctant veggie-eaters into increasing their veggie intakes with my Spicy Slaws as they add a new and interesting kick to raw or cooked veg. I love spice, so these recipes do contain generous amounts of pepper and chilli, but feel free to adapt the quantities if you like things to be slightly more 'relaxed'. Spicy Slaws are great for colder days, and Asian flavours impart a little warming sunshine. Many of the spices included in these recipes contain a special ingredient known as capsaicin, the chemical that is said to stimulate the natural process where the food we eat at each meal is converted immediately to heat.

If you don't have fresh chilli to hand, fear not! A few shakes of dried chilli flakes at the end or some pickled chilli from a jar will also add a little extra fire.

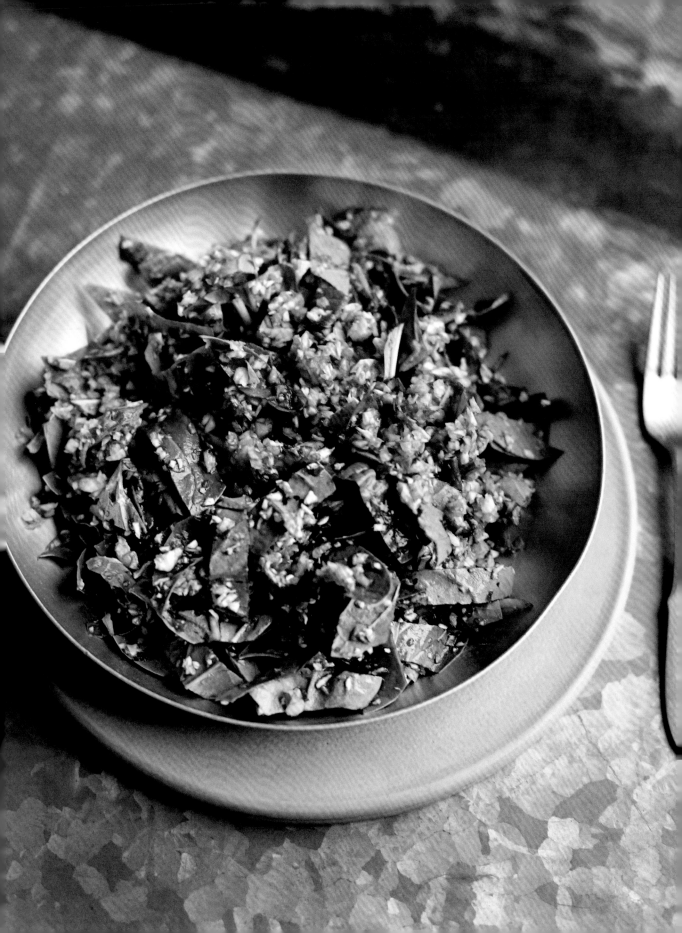

Smoky Pepper Slaw

Peppers are known to contain a compound called capsaicin, which studies have shown in large amounts can have a positive impact on raising the metabolism. Peppers are also super high in vitamins (A, B6 and C), so I love this as a winter warmer too if colds and flu are lurking.

If you need to sweeten things a little, just add a dash of tomato purée into the mix.

4 mixed red peppers (I use 2 small sweet peppers and 2 large), deseeded and any core removed
½ small red onion
½ teaspoon smoked paprika
½ teaspoon smoked chilli (I use it straight from a jar)
Splash of balsamic vinegar
Splash of olive oil
½ medium sweet cabbage, core removed and chopped into quarters
4–5 handfuls of spinach
Sea salt
Dash of tomato purée (optional)

Makes 4 large portions

1 Place the peppers, onion, paprika and chilli into the main bowl of the food processor with the central chopping attachment and pulse until similar to a paste.

2 Stir in the balsamic and olive oil and place in a waiting bowl.

3 Repeat by adding in the cabbage and pulse until a chunky chop. Add to the bowl.

4 Whizz the spinach in the food processor or shred by tearing or chopping with a knife.

5 Mix all of the ingredients together and stir, then taste and season. Add in a dash of tomato purée if you prefer the mixture a little sweeter.

toppers

Shredded roast beef.

morph your slaw

Baked Aubergine with Smoky Pepper Slaw

1 Slow bake 2 aubergines whole at 180°C for 45–60 minutes or until cooked through (the flesh should be mushy).

2 Scoop out of the aubergine flesh and mix into any leftover slaw.

3 Pan-fry the mixture for 1–2 minutes.

4 Top with chopped tomatoes and shredded beef.

Night of Passion Slaw

Adding a little spice to a night of passion will always be a winning combo!

Garam masala is a crushed mix of warming spices common in Asian cuisine. As convenience is the name of the game with SuperSlaw, I use the pre-mixed version (found in the spice section of most supermarkets).

The word 'garam' refers to the Ayurvedic meaning of 'heat of the body', and within the Ayurvedic medical system reference to these spices elevating the body's temperature as a means to raise metabolism and eliminate toxins is common among practioners.

6–8 stalks of celery, sliced into
   quarters
1 bag (50 g) of pea shoots
3 small heads of fennel, ends
   cut off
1 large handful of mint
2 passion fruit
Drizzle of olive oil
½ lemon
4 heaped tablespoons natural
   yoghurt
1 teaspoon garam masala
Sea salt

Makes 4 large portions

1 Place the celery and pea shoots into the main bowl of the food processor with the central chopping attachment and pulse until finely chopped. Add to a waiting bowl.

2 Repeat with the fennel and mint. Mix into the celery and pea shoots.

3 Cut the passion fruit into halves, scoop out the seeds using a spoon and add to a jam jar. Discard any red pith and the outer shell.

4 Add the olive oil, lemon juice, yoghurt and garam masala to the jar, replace the lid and shake vigorously until the mix is no longer separated. Add extra olive oil if needed.

5 Pour over the mixture, sprinkle with sea salt and mix well.

toppers

Steam a few handfuls of spinach and top your slaw with some extra iron.

morph your slaw

Pan-fried Paneer with Night of Passion Slaw

1 Cube a block of paneer cheese and pan-fry until cooked through, about 8 minutes.

2 Throw in any slaw and heat for 1–2 minutes.

3 Serve with steamed rice.

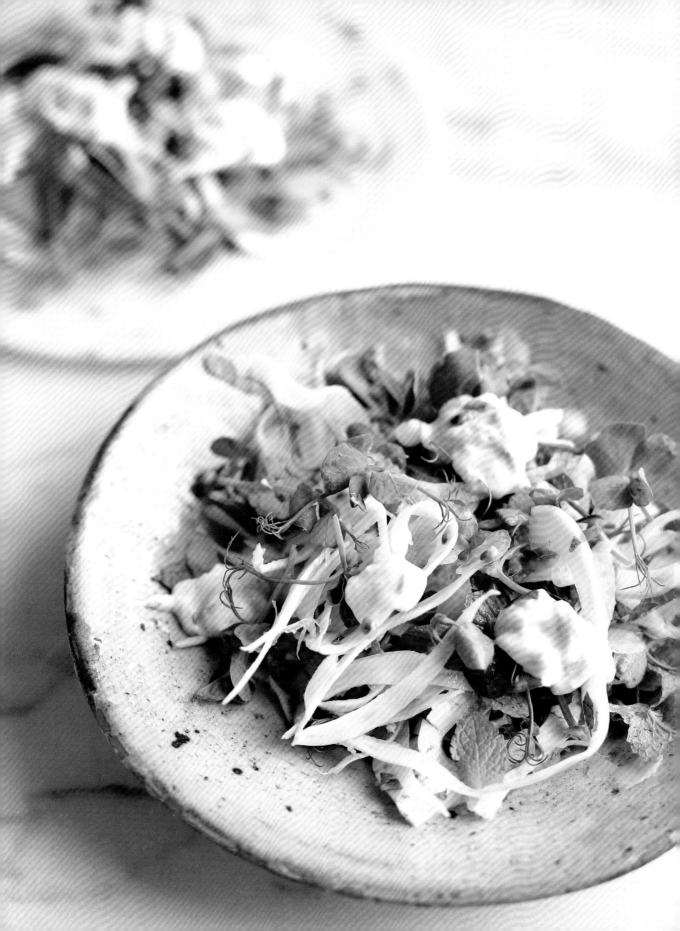

Thai Fragrant Slaw

Thai spice mixes and herbs can usually be bought pre-packed in supermarkets, which saves too much thinking time as to what flavours will work together. Medicinally lemongrass is a bit of a Thai wonder herb with reported benefits from increased relaxation to improved blood circulation! Whatever the truth behind this is, there is no doubt that Thai spices have a warming effect on the body and soul. The flavours in this slaw are subtle with a lovely Thai fragrance for the vegetables, so as a 'dry slaw' this tends to last longer throughout the week – perfect for a lunch box prep.

½ celeriac, peeled and chopped into sixths
4 carrots, peeled
8 baby corn
2 cm cube of galangal, peeled
2 stalks of lemongrass, peeled and trimmed
1 garlic clove, peeled
1 bird's-eye chilli, deseeded
Dash of light soy sauce (I use reduced-sodium)
3–4 tablespoons olive oil

Makes 4 large portions

TOPPER pictured

1 Place the celeriac pieces into the main section of the food processor with the central chopping attachment and pulse until they form small, even chopped pieces. Place into a waiting bowl.
2 Repeat, adding in any leftover celeriac pieces, the carrots and finally the baby corn.
3 Add the galangal, lemongrass, garlic and chilli to the food processor (alternatively, hand-chop). Blitz together until finely chopped. Remove any stalky pieces of lemongrass and dispose, then add the soy sauce and olive oil.
4 Mix all of the vegetables together.
5 Pour any extra olive oil, if needed, over the mix and mix well.

toppers

Cooked mixed seafood, fresh parsley leaves and a few wedges of lime.

morph your slaw
Fragrant Thai Slaw Fried Rice

1 Boil some jasmine rice according to the packet instructions.
2 Mix in any leftover slaw.
3 Pan-fry until the vegetables are soft, then top with your choice of cooked mixed seafood.

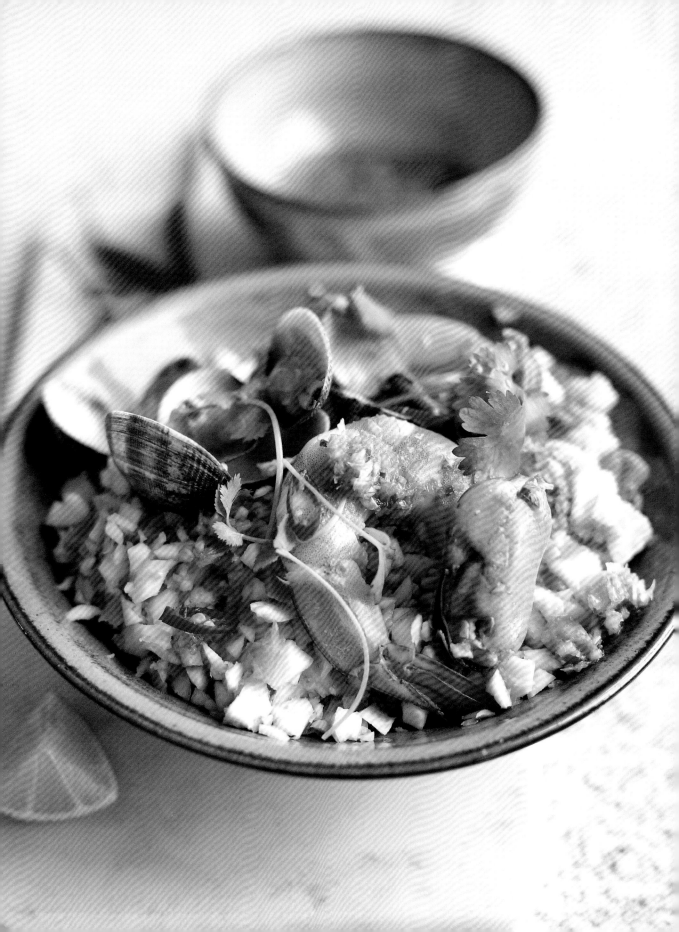

Luscious Lime Pickle 'Rice' Slaw

If you are the one at an Indian restaurant that likes to karate chop the poppadoms before nosediving into the pickles, then this is the slaw for you! Lime pickle is often served alongside milder or yoghurt-flavoured dips, so dependent on how brave you feel, you may want to go a little easy on the portion control in this slaw or check out the TOPPER to help cool things down. Lime pickle has a very strong flavour, so I like to use it just as a little taster alongside other fresher ingredients. If you aren't a fan of the sharp taste of the pickle, the recipe also works really well without it.

1 medium cauliflower, broken
　　into florets
1 large bunch of coriander
1 heaped tablespoon lime pickle
　　(optional)
1 green chilli, deseeded
2 limes, peel and deseed one and
　　halve the other
3–4 tablespoons olive oil
Sea salt
Dash of white wine vinegar
　　(optional)

Makes 4 large portions

1 Place the cauliflower florets into the main section of the food processor with the central chopping attachment and pulse until very finely chopped in a rice-like consistency. Add to a waiting bowl.

2 Repeat by blending most of the coriander (chopping and setting a little aside to garnish), the lime pickle, chilli and the peeled lime. Pour and mix into the cauliflower.

3 Add the olive oil and the juice from the remaining lime to a jam jar with a sprinkle of sea salt, replace the lid and shake vigorously. Add the vinegar if needed.

4 Pour over the slaw and mix together well.

5 Garnish with the remaining chopped coriander.

toppers

A mix of Greek or natural yoghurt with a dash of mint will help cool things down!

morph your slaw
Cauliflower, Lime Pickle + Tomato Curry

1 Pan-fry any leftover slaw for a few minutes until lightly cooked.

2 Pour over a 400g tin of chopped tomatoes and heat through for a couple of minutes.

3 Serve with chicken or a protein of your choice.

Choi Sum Slaw

Sweet tooth? A great tip for anyone who suffers with regular sweet cravings – try and eat something salty first and see if your craving changes.

Salty and pickled flavours are great for curbing a sweet tooth. You can play around with the chilli content of this recipe a little. If I feel like an extra bit of heat, I may swap the green chilli for the hotter red version, giving it a little extra boost. I fell in love with choi sum on my travels to Hong Kong, where so many dishes have this as a staple. Supplying the perfect combo of vitamin C and iron, it adds a lovely unusual flavour. If you can't track it down, feel free to swap for any other Asian leaves.

1 bag (150–200 g) of dark leafy cabbage leaves
1 bag (150–200 g) of choi sum (if you struggle to source this, it can be replaced with pak choi)
¼ jar capers, drained
½ jar mini gherkins
2 green chillies, deseeded
Drizzle of olive oil
2–4 tablespoons white balsamic vinegar
Few dashes of soy sauce (I use reduced-sodium)
½ teaspoon cayenne pepper

Makes 4 large portions

1 Place the central chopping attachment into the main bowl of the food processor.
2 Place the cabbage and choi sum into the bowl and gently pulse until chopped. Tip into a waiting bowl.
3 Next, add the capers, gherkins and chillies to the food processor. Blend until they form small, chunky pieces. They will go a little mushy. Add to a waiting jam jar.
4 Add the olive oil, vinegar, soy and cayenne pepper to the jam jar. Place the lid on and shake vigorously. Pour over the slaw and mix well.

toppers
Add a little wild garlic

morph your slaw
Stir-fry Choi Sum Slaw with Ginger + Garlic

1 Heat a little oil in a pan and add minced garlic and chopped ginger. Cook for a few minutes.
2 Add any leftover slaw and cook for 2–3 minutes.

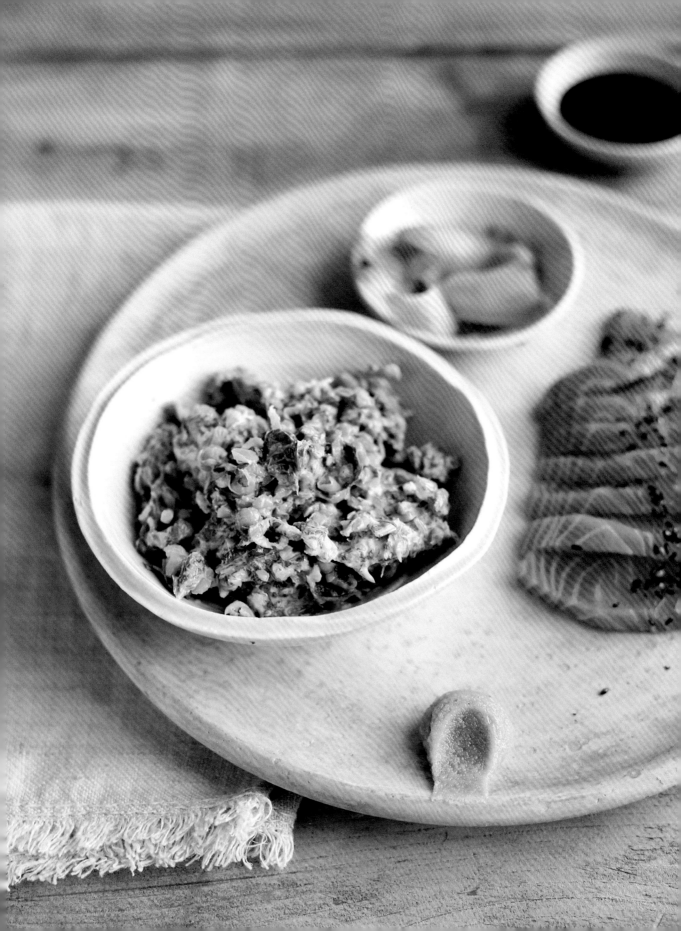

Wasabi Slaw

Wasabi is a Japanese plant from the horseradish family, most readily available either in a powder or a paste form (although check the packet for authenticity – there are many 'fake' wasabi products out there with very little actual wasabi in them). If you are a newcomer to the world of this magical spice, then be warned, wasabi is not for the faint-hearted! Japanese researchers even won an award for the development of wasabi as a means to awaken and alert people in the event of an emergency.

1 small bag (250 g) of frozen peas, slightly defrosted by placing in cold water, then draining
1 bag (150 g) of sugar snap peas
1 bag (150 g) of rocket leaves
1 heaped tablespoon crème fraîche or Greek yoghurt
2 tablespoons rice wine vinegar
1 heaped tablespoon wasabi
Splash of light soy sauce (I use reduced-sodium)
Splash of white wine vinegar

Makes 4 large portions

MORPH pictured

1 Place the frozen peas into the main section of the food processor with the central chopping attachment and pulse until they form small, evenly chopped pieces (stop just before it creates a mushy consistency). Place into a waiting bowl.

2 Repeat by adding the sugar snaps and rocket leaves to the processor. Mix into the frozen peas.

3 Add the crème fraîche, rice wine vinegar, wasabi and soy to a jam jar. Replace the lid and shake vigorously. Pour the thick mixture over the veg and mix well.

4 Pour the splash of white wine vinegar into the bottom of the jar and use this to thin and clean out any remaining mixture. Pour over the slaw and mix together well.

toppers

Grated or pickled ginger.

morph your slaw
Wasabi Sashimi

1 Place some sliced good-quality raw fish (you can ask your local fishmonger what fish is freshest for this) on a plate.

2 Add scoops of leftover slaw, slices of pickled ginger, soy sauce and wasabi.

Ginger Fire Slaw

Mooli looks a little like a giant white carrot, but is a member of the horseradish family and is now regularly found in the Asian vegetable section of most supermarkets. It works really well with pickled flavours. Adding a little plum TOPPER to the mix creates a beautifully fresh, but fiery fruity-flavoured slaw. This recipe is also loaded with heaps of ginger. Ginger is said to be a 'vasodilator', which basically means it enhances circulation of the blood, increasing body temperature and promoting metabolic benefits!

*1 large mooli, peeled and cut into
    quarters*
6 stalks of celery, cut into quarters
*2 tablespoons pickled jalapeño
    peppers*
*1 large cube (about 2 cm) of fresh
    ginger*
2–3 tablespoons olive oil
2 tablespoons Worcestershire sauce
Sea salt

Makes 4 large portions

TOPPER pictured

1 Place the mooli into the main bowl of the food processor with the central chopping attachment and pulse until it forms chunky chopped pieces.
2 Repeat, by adding in the celery and jalapeno peppers, then pour and mix into the mooli.
3 Grate the ginger into the mix and stir.
4 Add the olive oil, Worcestershire sauce and a sprinkle of sea salt to a jam jar, replace the lid and shake vigorously. Add any vinegar if needed.
5 Pour over the mix. Mix well.

toppers

Fire up your plums by adding them as a TOPPER to your slaw.

morph your slaw

Shredded Duck + Hot Ginger Fire Salad

1 Coat a duck breast in a little salt and five spice powder. Roast in a 220°C oven for 20 minutes until cooked through and crispy.
2 Shred once cool enough to handle.
3 Pour any duck juices into a pan and fry any leftover slaw for 1–2 minutes.
4 Serve with the duck and slices of plum.

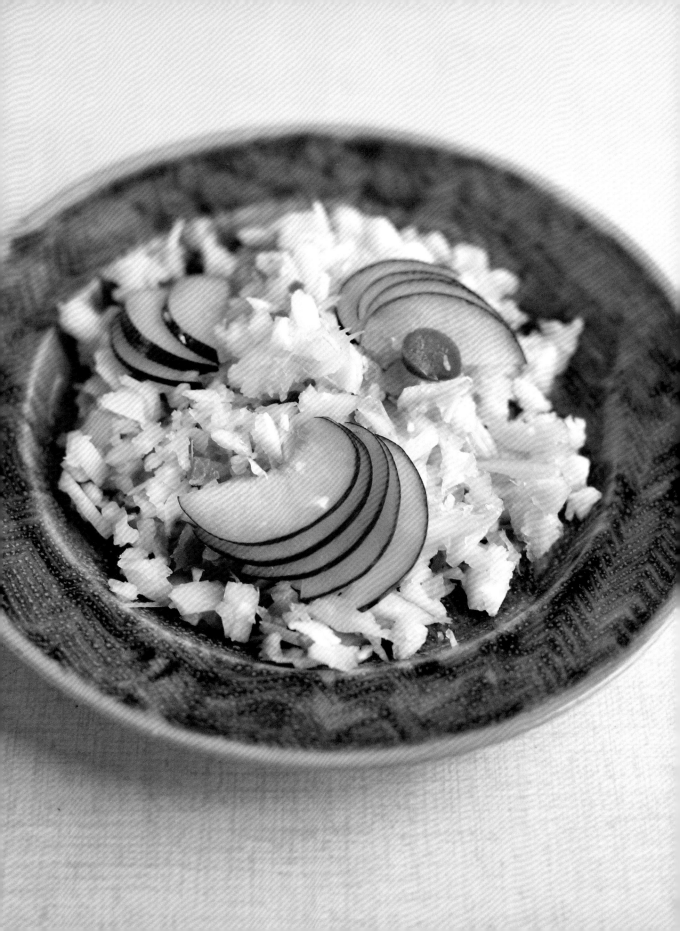

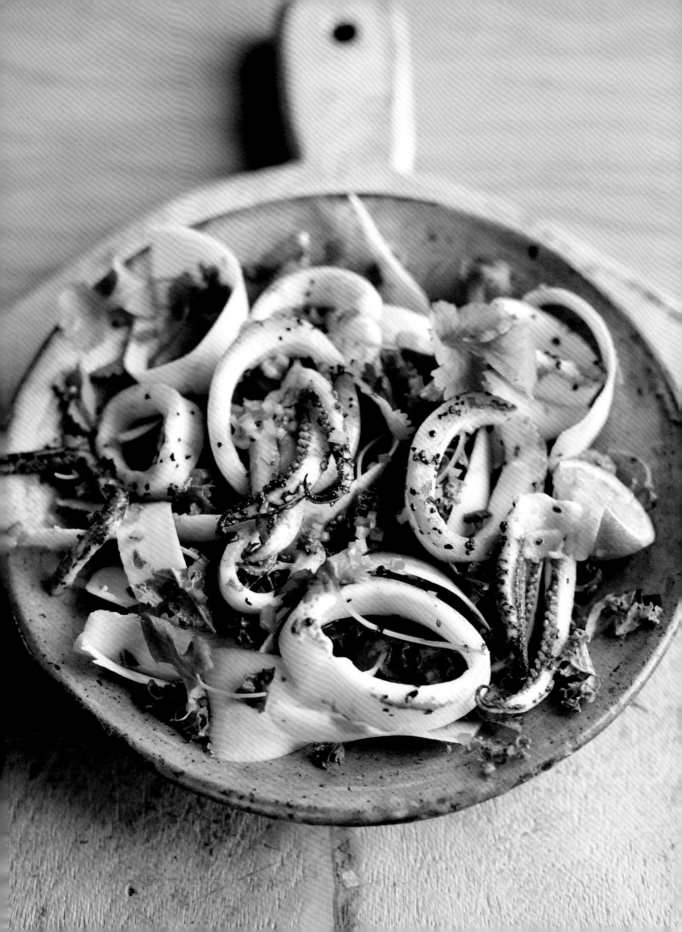

Spice Kick Slaw

This is a great slaw for when you feel you need a bit of a warming boost. In the winter I suffer with poor circulation (especially after training clients outdoors in the delights of the Manchester weather), so I like to add fire into my meals to help me feel more alive again. I really enjoy the texture of parsnip shavings so I peel these into the mix, but you can always add to the food processor if you have less time.

200 g kale
6 large gherkins
3 large parsnips, peeled
1 green chilli, deseeded and sliced
1 red chilli, deseeded and sliced
1 cube of fresh ginger, peeled
2–3 handfuls of coriander
1 lime, halved
Drizzle of olive oil
2–3 tablespoons balsamic vinegar
Sea salt

Makes 4 large portions

MORPH pictured

1 Place the kale and the gherkins into the main bowl of the food processor with the central chopping attachment and pulse until finely chopped. Add to a waiting bowl.

2 Peel in the parsnips using a potato peeler. This is a little time consuming, but is worth it I promise. Alternatively, use the food processor.

3 Hand-chop the chillies and ginger into fine slices and mix in with the chopped vegetables.

4 Roughly chop the coriander and mix in.

5 Squeeze the juice of the lime over the mix.

6 Mix the olive oil and vinegar in a jam jar. Pour over the slaw.

7 Season with sea salt and mix well.

toppers

Fried courgette pieces make a great TOPPER.

morph your slaw

Salt + Pepper Squid Spice Kick

1 Season some raw squid pieces with a good helping of salt and pepper.

2 Chargrill on a very hot grill until cooked, about 1 minute on each side.

3 Serve mixed into any leftover slaw.

Indian Street Slaw

Indian flavours are often complex. Making traditional Indian food can take a lot of time and patience to master. This slaw allows you to feel as though you've indulged in a little Indian creativity without spending hours in the kitchen. Even better than that, you get to feel guilt free about having a curry! If you feel extra virtuous, you can add a little fresh mango to this dish in exchange for the chutney — thereby lowering the sugar content.

2 carrots, peeled and topped
10 radishes, topped and tailed
10 stalks of celery
1 red chilli, deseeded
2 handfuls (roughly 150 g) of
    coriander
1 handful (roughly 75 g) of mint
2 little gem lettuces (or 3 if very
    small)
2 tablespoons olive oil
1 tablespoon mango chutney
1 handful of fresh or dried curry
    leaves
1 lemon, halved
Sea salt

Makes 4 large portions

1 Place the central chopping attachment into the main bowl of the food processor and add the carrots and radishes. Pulse until chopped (they are dense vegetables so may take a little longer to chop). Add to a waiting bowl.

2 Now add the celery, chilli and fresh herbs. Pulse until chopped and add to the vegetables.

3 Shred the gem lettuce by roughly chopping with a knife into thick strips. Mix with the rest of the ingredients in the waiting bowl.

4 Add the olive oil, chutney and curry leaves to a jam jar. Place the lid on and shake vigorously. Add to the slaw. Squeeze over the juice of the lemon, sprinkle with sea salt and mix well.

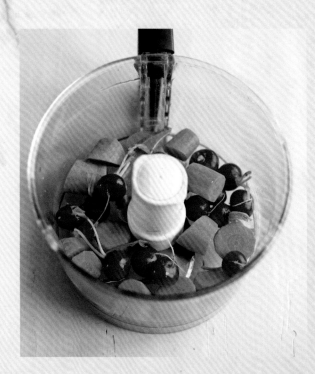

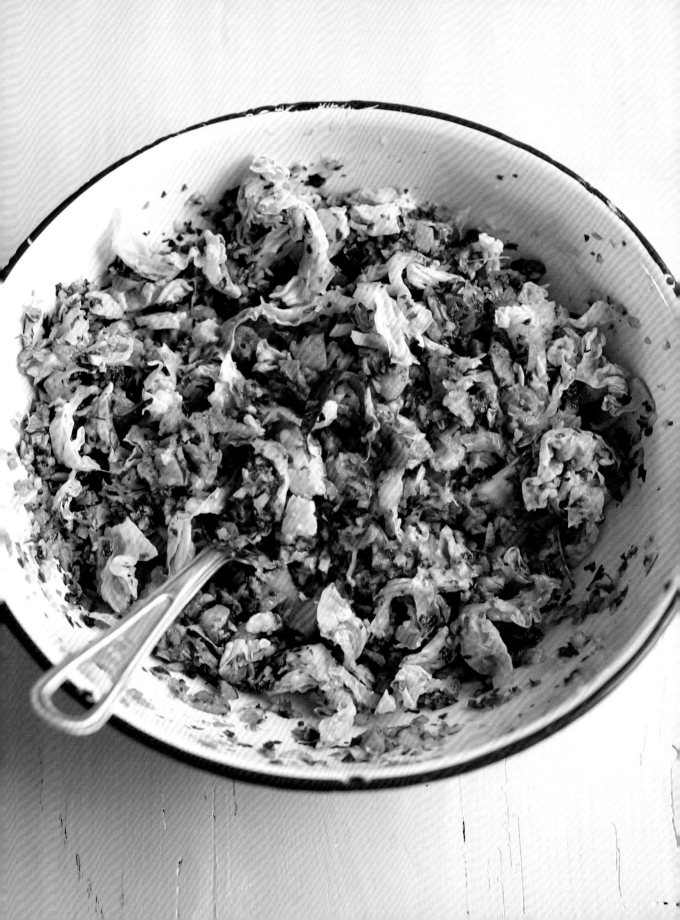

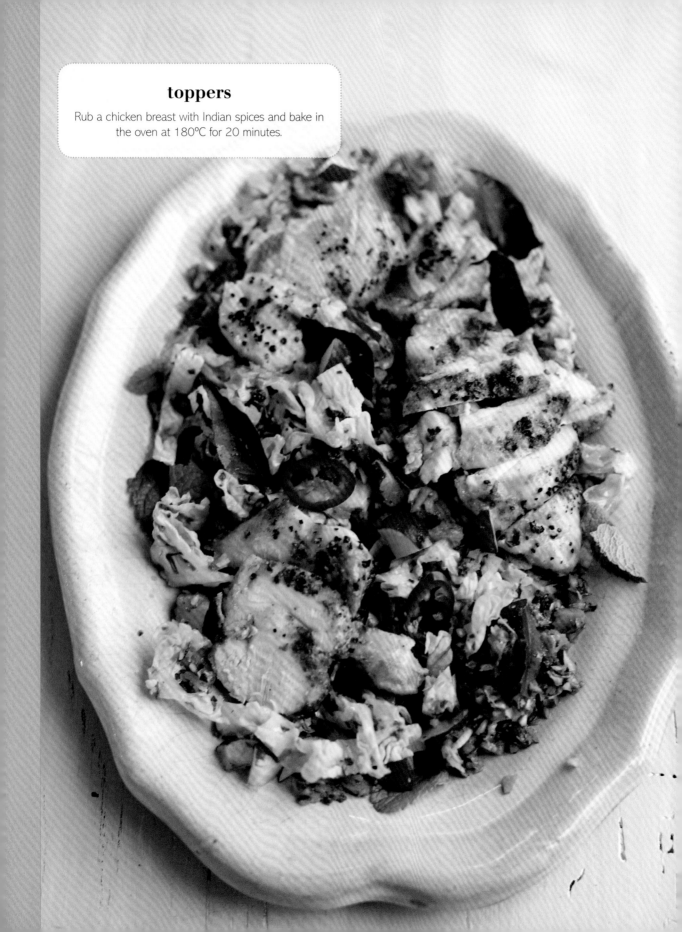

toppers

Rub a chicken breast with Indian spices and bake in the oven at 180°C for 20 minutes.

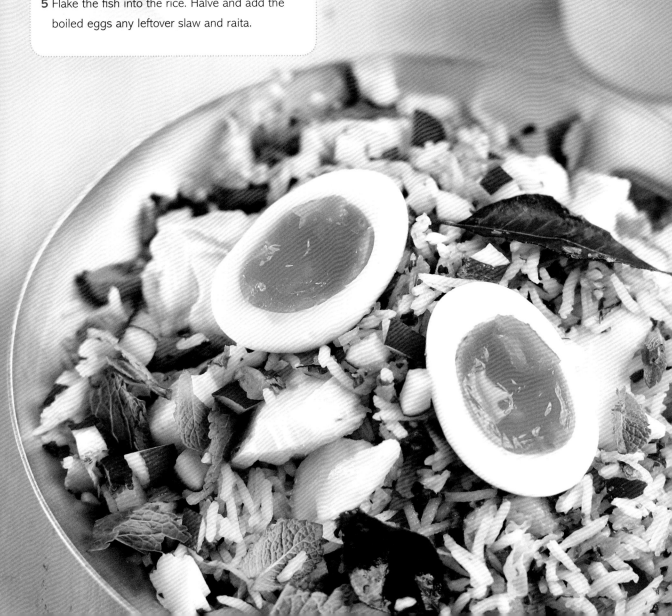

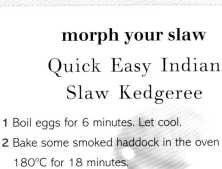

morph your slaw

Quick Easy Indian
Slaw Kedgeree

1 Boil eggs for 6 minutes. Let cool.

2 Bake some smoked haddock in the oven at 180°C for 18 minutes.

3 Cook white basmati rice according to the packet instructions.

4 Mix together a quick-and-easy raita by stirring together natural yoghurt, mint and cumin.

5 Flake the fish into the rice. Halve and add the boiled eggs any leftover slaw and raita.

Asian Cabbage Slaw

Asian Cabbage Slaw is the ultimate slaw MORPH as it tastes so different when you tackle this hot versus cold, so it's worth making this one in bulk if you want to try the variation. This slaw makes a light, but satiating change to a lunchtime salad. Adding rice noodles and a protein source, then topping with some spring onion shavings, will save you both money and the extra calories from nipping to the local takeaway!

1 small red cabbage, core remove and cut into sixths
1 small white cabbage, core removed and cut into sixths
5 large carrots, peeled
1 bag (150 g) of mangetout
3 large handfuls of coriander
4 limes, halved
2–3 tablespoons soy sauce (I use reduced-sodium)
2–3 tablespoons fish sauce
2–3 tablespoons toasted sesame seeds
½ teaspoon ground cinnamon

Makes 4 large portions

1 Place the red cabbage into the main bowl of the food processor with the central chopping attachment and pulse until it forms fine pieces. Add to a waiting bowl.
2 Repeat with the white cabbage and then the carrots. Mix all the vegetables together.
3 Hand-chop the mangetout into fine pieces and add to the mix.
4 Hand-chop the coriander and mix in.
5 Squeeze the juice of the limes over the mix.
6 Add the soy and fish sauces.
7 Sprinkle with the sesame seeds and cinnamon and mix well.

toppers

Shavings of spring onion.

morph your slaw
Stir-fried Prawns with Asian Slaw

1 Heat some rice noodles by pouring over some boiling water for 2–3 minutes. Drain.
2 Pan-fry some prawns until cooked, about 2 minutes. Add in the slaw and heat through.
3 Serve mixed with the rice noodles.

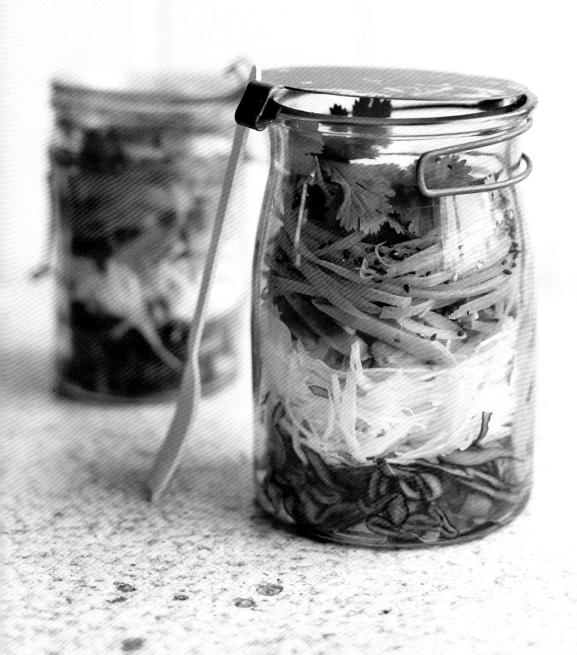

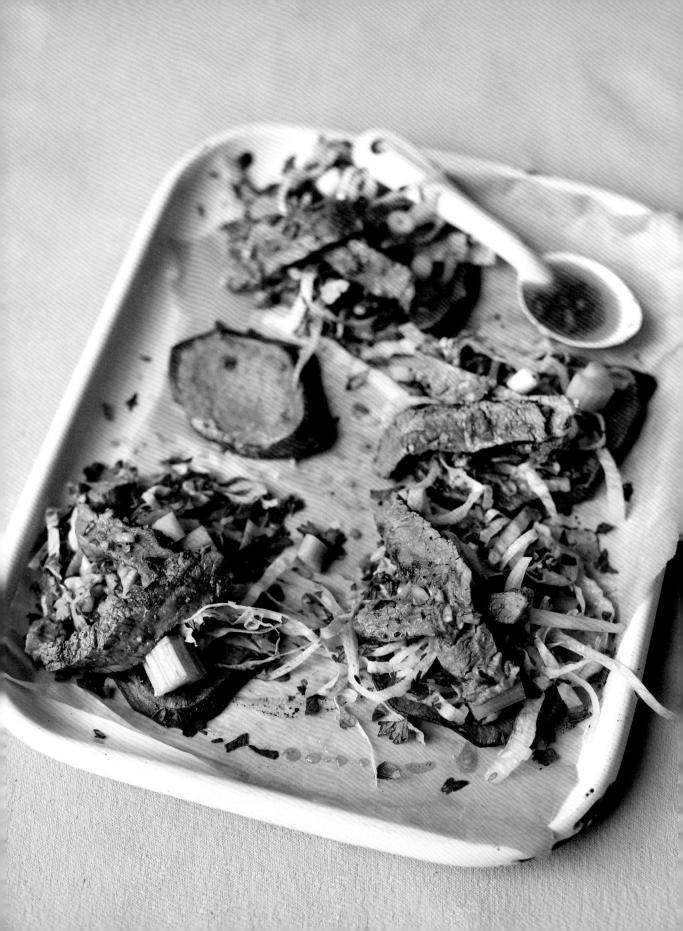

Chimichurri Slaw

Chimichurri is a fiery flavour, typically associated with Argentinian dishes. Paprika is made from ground capsicums, so this is a perfect spice for giving the metabolism a little peak. A tiny sprinkle here and there not only adds a warming boost, but also provides good amounts of vitamins A, E, B and iron. I have suggested a fresh mango TOPPER in this recipe to add a little hint of fruit at the end, but for an alternative option try adding dried mango pieces into the food processor.

200 g parsley
6 stalks of celery
2 spring onions
2–3 handfuls of iceberg lettuce
2 baby shallots
1 garlic clove, peeled
3–4 tablespoons olive oil
3–4 tablespoons red wine vinegar
Pinch of dried oregano
½ teaspoon smoked paprika
Pinch of chilli powder
Sea salt

Makes 4 large portions

MORPH pictured

1 Place the parsley into the main bowl of the food processor with the central chopping attachment and pulse until small pieces form (you may have to do this in batches). Place in a waiting bowl.

2 Repeat with the celery and spring onions and chop until they form chunkily chopped pieces. Mix into the parsley.

3 Repeat the above with the iceberg lettuce and mix in (alternatively, you can finely shred with a knife).

4 Hand-chop the shallots and garlic into fine pieces. Place in a waiting jam jar.

5 Place the olive oil, vinegar, oregano, spices and a sprinkle of sea salt into the jar with the shallots and garlic. Replace the lid and shake vigorously.

6 Pour the thick mixture over the veg and mix well.

toppers

Fresh mango slices.

morph your slaw
Chimichurri Steak with Sweet Potato

1 Bake slices of sweet potato drizzled with a little oil in a 180°C oven and cook for about 20 minutes or until crispy.

2 Meanwhile, pan-fry a steak until just pink in the middle, about 3 minutes on each side. Place on a board to rest for a few minutes.

4 Slice the steak into strips and place on top of the leftover slaw. Serve.

Additional Recommendations for Macronutrients

Nutrients are substances needed by the body for a huge variation of tasks, including growth, repair, energy production and many other bodily functions. However, the amounts needed by the body varies. Nutrients can be divided into two main headings:

Micronutrients + Macronutrients

Micronutrients include both fat-soluble and water soluble vitamins, minerals and water. They are needed in small amounts by the body. No single food contains all the vitamins and minerals you need, so a balanced and varied diet is necessary. You will find a wide array of micronutrients in every SuperSlaw.

Macronutrients, on the other hand, are required in greater amounts and can be seen as the three main or key substances needed by humans. They are generally categorized or separated into protein, carbohydrates and fats.

Macronutrient and micronutrient requirements vary from person to person and can be influenced by a number of both genetic and lifestyle factors.

Macronutrients provide calories (or energy) to the body in different amounts. Carbohydrates and protein, for example, provide 4 calories per gram, conversely fat provides a higher figure at 9 calories per gram.

To ensure a full combination of macronutrients, I have included suggested TOPPERS and MORPHS within every recipe based on a range of fats, proteins and carbohydrates. However, as I am a huge advocate of a creative approach when you combine each SuperSlaw, then I'd also love for you to try experimenting with other macronutrients, right:

Protein

Protein is an essential macronutrient, fairly well known as being related to muscle maintenance and growth. Due to this it holds a pivotal place in metabolic health. Protein is multifunctional, so in addition to aiding metabolism, it also helps the body in other areas including gut health. It is highly recommended as holding a regular place on every plate. Along with fibre-rich foods, protein also helps to keep you full. Try and vary your sources of protein as much as possible to achieve a diversity of amino acids. Below are a list of good-quality protein sources you can experiment with as alternatives to those provided within the recipe recommendations:

Fish

Seafood

Poultry

Eggs

Red meat

Game

Quinoa

Tofu

Mixed beans and peas

Chickpeas

Soy beans, pulses and lentils

Carbohydrates

Carbohydrates are a macronutrient that invokes a huge range of nutritional opinion. They are technically non-essential, although trying to go long periods of time without them is not something I would recommend for most people (without medical or dietician supervision or advice). Carbohydrates are unbeatable for the use of high-energy production, so if you want changes to body composition along with success in fitness performance, in my experience most people gain more progress with carbohydrates in their diets. Below are a list of carbohydrate sources that you can experiment with as alternatives to those provided within the recipe recommendations:

- Sweet potato
- New potato
- Butternut squash
- Basmati rice
- Jasmine rice
- Wild rice
- Quinoa
- Mixed whole grains
- Rye bread
- Other root vegetables that may require cooking (turnip/swede, etc.)

Fat

Fat has developed a bad reputation over the years, thanks to the low-calorie, low-fat diet lovers. And there is no question that fat is the most calorie-dense nutrient.

However, a common failure of many low-fat diet plans comes down to their lack of fat. The body cannot function well without fats. This is where you will have heard the phrase 'essential fats'. These essential fatty acids (omega 3 + 6) are vital for growth and development and for the proper functioning of our nerves and brain. The body also needs fat to absorb vital nutrients. Without fat to aid this process, with all the good will (or green superfood plans) in the world, nutrients will simply be wasted.

Main point to take away: the body needs fat to absorb the good stuff from the slaw. If you cut your fat too much, you cut your vitamin absorption potential by default. This is why I encourage olive oil to be used in most of the recipes.

Examples of some extra fats that can be added to your SuperSlaw, either as a TOPPER, dressing or side dish:

- Coconut oil and/or fresh coconut
- Organic butter
- Animal fat (through meat)
- Olive oil/other natural oils
- Avocado
- Olives
- Oily fish especially salmon, mackerel and sardines
- Nuts
- Seeds

Index

A

allotment slaw 57
anchovies: stuffed
    peppers with anchovies
    + salsa slaw 97
apples: applephire slaw 61
    sweet + sour apple
    slaw 131
Asian cabbage slaw 152
asparagus: ham
    asparagus vit-kick rolls
    46
aubergines: baked
    aubergine with smoky
    pepper slaw 135
avocados: avocado kale
    slaw 85
    broc-a-mole slaw 82

B

bacon: tutti-frutti bacon
    salad 121
bake, creamy cauliflower,
    feta & tomato 81
basil: pesto punch slaw 69
    watercress, beans +
    basil slaw 37
    watermelon + basil
    slaw 125
bean sprouts, stir-fried
    purple power with 58
beef: chimichurri steak
    with sweet potato 155
    hot steak superslaw
    salad 48
beetroot: beetroot blast
    slaw 126
    purple punch slaw 117
blueberries: frozen
    blueberry + egg salad
    41
broccoli: broc-a-mole
    slaw 82
    pineapple + purple
    broccoli slaw 63
    purple power slaw 58
    purple punch slaw 117
burgers, sweet potato

pesto 69

C

cabbage: Asian cabbage
    slaw 152
carbohydrates 157
cashew nuts: pesto
    punch slaw 69
cauliflower: cauliflower
    feta slaw 78
    creamy cauliflower, feta
    & tomato bake 81
    luscious lime pickle
    'rice' slaw 140
celeriac slaw 103
cheese: creamy
    cauliflower, feta &
    tomato bake 81
    fresh + pickle slaw 91
    green Greek omelette
    54
    pan fried paneer with
    night of passion slaw
    136
    roasted plum + goat's
    cheese smoothie slaw
    64
    ruby green cheese slaw
    32
chicken: honey + sesame
    za'atar chicken 38
    purple punch couscous
    salad with chicken 117
chicory pear slaw 41
chillies: Iron Maiden hot
    salsa 47
    spicy Texas slaw 74
chimichurri slaw 155
chocolate protein nut
    smoothie bowl 70
choi sum slaw 141
chorizo: hot chorizo +
    baby potato slaw 128
coco-lime slaw 100
courgette, tomato +
    quark slaw 127
couscous: purple punch
    couscous salad with

chicken 117
crunchy slaw 48
cucumber: tzatziki slaw
    109
curry, cauliflower, lime
    pickle + tomato 140

D

duck: shredded duck + hot
    ginger fire salad 144

E

edamame beans:
    Japanese edamame
    slaw 122
eggs: frozen blueberry +
    egg salad 41
    green Greek omelette
    54
    quick easy Indian slaw
    kedgeree 151

F

fat 157
fennel slaw, fruity 92
fish: baked fish with
    potato applephire salad
    61
    easy cheesy pickle fish
    slaw cakes 91
    quick easy Indian slaw
    kedgeree 151
    sweet potato + lively
    lemon fish cakes 24
    tartare fish + seafood
    salad 28
    wasabi sashimi 143
    see also salmon; tuna,
    etc
fresh + minty slaw 34
fresh + pickle slaw 91
fresh + simple slaw 29
fruit: fruity fennel slaw 92
    superhero fruit salad 94

G

ginger: ginger fire slaw
    144

stir-fry choi sum slaw
    with ginger + garlic 141
go-go greens 52
green beans: watercress,
    beans + basil slaw 37
green garden slaw 87
green Greek omelette 54

H

ham asparagus vit-kick
    rolls 46
honey + sesame za'atar
    chicken 38
hummus slaw 77

I

Indian street slaw 148
Iron Maiden slaw 47

J

Japanese edamame slaw
    122

K

kale: avocado kale slaw
    85
kebabs, hummus 77
kedgeree, quick easy
    Indian slaw 151

L

lamb chop superslaw,
    Mediterranean 34
lemons: lively lemon slaw
    24
    tahini + lemon slaw 93
lettuce: iceberg tartare
    slaw 28
limes: coco-lime slaw 100
    luscious lime pickle
    'rice' slaw 140

M

mackerel: smoked
    mackerel beetroot blast
    126
    tahini + lemon slaw
    mash with mackerel 93

macronutrients 156–7
Mediterranean lamb chop superslaw 34
Mediterranean sunshine slaw 27
micronutrients 156–7
mint: fresh + minty slaw 34
pea + mint slaw 114
mustard: creamy watercress mustard slaw 37

N
night of passion slaw 136
noodles, peanut satay 84
nori tzatziki slaw wrap 109
nuts: nut butter fruity fennel 92
nuts about slaw 70

O
omelette, green Greek 54
onion slaw, sweet 56

P
pan-fry, creamy allotment quick 57
paneer: pan fried paneer with night of passion slaw 136
papaya slaw 110
Parma ham stuffed watermelon rolls 125
passion fruit: night of passion slaw 136
pea + mint slaw 114
peanut satay slaw 84
pears: chicory pear slaw 41
peppers: smoky pepper slaw 135
stuffed peppers with anchovies + salsa slaw 97
pesto punch slaw 69
pickles: fresh + pickle slaw 91
luscious lime pickle 'rice' slaw 140
pineapple + purple

broccoli slaw 63
pizza: pizza slaw 104
pizza wrap 106
quinoa crackle pizza 73
plums: roasted plum + goat's cheese smoothie slaw 64
potatoes: baby potato + red spring onion slaw 128
baked fish with potato applephire salad 61
stuffed potato skins 127
prawns: papaya prawn stir-fry 110
stir-fried prawns with Asian slaw 152
protein 156
Provence slaw 98
purple power slaw 58
purple punch slaw 117

Q
quark: courgette, tomato + quark slaw 127
quinoa: nuts about slaw 70
quinoa crackle slaw 73

R
rice: fragrant Thai slaw fried rice 138
Japanese layered rice salad 122
ruby green cheese slaw 32
ruby green slaw 30

S
salmon: chunky celeriac mash with salmon 103
salmon, pineapple + purple broccoli pita 63
salsa: Iron Maiden hot salsa 47
salsa slaw 97
salt + pepper squid spice kick 147
samphire: applephire slaw 61
sashimi, wasabi 143

satay slaw, peanut 84
seafood: tartare fish + seafood salad 28
smoothie bowl, chocolate protein nut 70
soups: coco-lime-coco soup 100
pea + mint soup 114
spice kick slaw 147
spicy Texas slaw 74
spinach: avocado kale spinach wrap 85
spring onions: baby potato + red spring onion slaw 128
squid: salt + pepper squid spice kick 147
stir-fries: baby turnip fire + tofu stir-fry 51
papaya prawn stir-fry 110
stir-fried prawns with Asian slaw 152
stir-fried purple power with bean sprouts 58
stir-fry choi sum slaw with ginger + garlic 141
super-smoothie-Tasha slaw 64
superhero slaw 94
sweet + sour apple slaw 131
sweet potatoes: broc-a-mole creamy sweet potato wedges 82
chimichurri steak with sweet potato 155
sweet potato + lively lemon fish cakes 24
sweet potato pesto burgers 69

T
tahini + lemon slaw 93
tartare fish + seafood salad 28
Texas chilli 74
Texas slaw, spicy 74
Thai fragrant slaw 138
tofu: baby turnip fire + tofu stir-fry 51

roasted vegetable garden slaw with tofu 87
tomatoes: cauliflower, lime pickle + tomato curry 140
courgette, tomato + quark slaw 127
creamy cauliflower, feta & tomato bake 81
Iron Maiden hot salsa 47
trout, baked sweet onion 56
tuna: fresh + simple tuna salad twist 29
turkey: minced sweet + spicy turkey fry 131
turnips: baby turnip fire slaw 51
tutti-frutti bacon salad 121
tutti-frutti slaw 118
tzatziki slaw 109

V
vegetables: baked Mediterranean vegetable slaw 27
roasted vegetable garden slaw with tofu 87
vit-kick rolls, ham asparagus 46
vit-kick slaw 45

W
wasabi slaw 143
watercress, beans + basil slaw 37
watermelon + basil slaw 125
wraps: avocado kale spinach wrap 85
nori tzatziki slaw wrap 109
pizza wrap 106

Y
yoghurt: tzatziki slaw 109

Z
za'atar slaw 38

Dedicated to

With love to the ultimate + original 'SUPER GREENS' – Mum, Dad and all of the Greenwood family.

To Iron Man Ash – for all of the love and all of the coffee (I am blessed to have so much of both) x

Acknowledgements

So many 'super' people to thank for their support and inspiration within my SuperSlaw journey:

To my incredible agents Graham Maw Christie – Jen, you are simply brilliant. Thank you for encouraging me, and believing in my vision every step of the way. To Juliette T and Mark W, for persuading me to initially go for it – it is thanks to you that I did — and to Nathan for all things web-site'y' and for preventing me from throwing my Mac out of the window. To JWM for being bored to tears with my grammar, and Carolyn for teaching me many years ago how to dress a salad with a jam jar.

To Lisa, Louise, Kay and Barbara and all of the team at Ebury and Penguin Random House. And to the styling and photo superstars, Lara, Frankie and Sophie – I feel truly quite privileged to have worked with the best and the loveliest in the business.

To my parents who have taught me the never-ending lesson of persistence at times when life gives you a challenge. To Sharon, Denise, Paul and their respective families – thank you for supporting every inch of my creative (and often unconventional) plans in life, even when this means eating SuperSlaw on Christmas day.

To all those on my strength journey (Andy Coach Rimmer, Ged O'hara and my kettlebellwarrior clients), high-five for keeping me physically strong in both body + mind. To my girlfriends (near and far) – you know who you are, thank you for tirelessly supporting me becoming a bit of a work bore, and coping with vegetables now being my main topic of conversation. Super huge thank you to every social media request and shout out for my recipes, I hope this doesn't disappoint. A big thank you to the staff at the Didsbury Lounge, who have kept me beautifully hydrated, ok 'caffeinated', throughout 95% of this manuscript.

Last but by no means least, to the Iron Man in my life, Ash, who has been both chief critic and tester for every SuperSlaw, and has managed to keep his patience at times when the kitchen sink began to resemble an unruly vegetable tip. Thank you for having superhero status in my life, (even with slaw stuck between your toes).

Follow Me on:
Twitter: www.twitter.com/@jillkbw
Instagram: www.instagram.com/jillgreenwood/
FaceBook: www.facebook.com/JillGreenwood.co.uk/